SIRENS AND STORIES

AN ANTHOLOGY OF THE PARAMEDIC PROFESSION

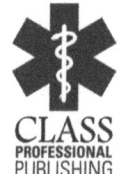

CLASS
PROFESSIONAL
PUBLISHING

Text © Georgette Eaton 2024.

All rights reserved. Without limiting the rights under copyright reserved above, no part of this publication may be reproduced, stored in or introduced into a retrieval system, or transmitted, in any form or by any means (electronic, mechanical, photocopying, recording or otherwise) without the prior written permission of the publisher of this book.

Disclaimer:
This collection of short stories and poems is inspired by real events; however, names, characters, places and incidents have been altered or fictionalised to protect the privacy and anonymity of the individuals involved. Any resemblance to actual persons, living or dead, or actual events is purely coincidental.

Printing history:
This first edition published in 2024.

The authors and publisher welcome feedback from the users of this book. Please contact the publisher:

Class Professional Publishing,
The Exchange, Express Park, Bristol Road, Bridgwater TA6 4RR

Telephone: 01278 472 800
Email: info@class.co.uk
Website: www.classprofessional.co.uk

Class Professional Publishing is an imprint of Class Publishing Ltd.
A CIP catalogue record for this book is available from the British Library.

Paperback ISBN: 9781801610544
ePUB ISBN: 9781801610551
ePDF ISBN: 9781801610568

Cover design by Nicky Borowiec
Designed and typeset by PHi Business Solutions
Printed in the UK by Ashford Colour Press Ltd

This book is printed on paper from responsible sources. Refer to local recycling guidance on disposal of this book.

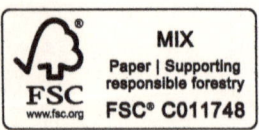

CONTENTS

Foreword   ix
Jules Swain

Preface   xi
Georgette Eaton

Day Shift

Provided that   2
Lawrence Hill

The lament of a student paramedic   4
Carrie Martin

Welcome to the ambulance service   5
Sarah Hennessy

Rats of the sky   7
Richard Green

You did your job   8
Anonymous

Are you the ambulance driver?   9
Emma Chetwood

Biceps blues: a shower saga   11
Ashley Lucas

A nose for trouble   13
Sarah-Jane Niles

Sprain   17
Monica Thompson

Sneeze-on   17
Monica Thompson

Zombie chicken pox   17
Monica Thompson

The unlikely asylum seekers *Lucy McKenzie*	18
Bedside intruders *Sarah-Jane Niles*	21
A job that took us by surprise *Lucy McKenzie*	24
Another life saved *Anonymous*	28
Memories *Neil Armstrong*	34
More than medicine *Gemma Butler*	36
Around the mess table *Karen Scott*	38
Naji (Survivor) *Iain Campbell*	39
Stepping into advanced practice *Jared Gooch*	42
My father's legacy *Nick Williams*	45
Not the rollercoaster you thought *Anonymous*	46
Intuition *Caroline French*	48
Keeping in touch *Charlie McCourt*	50
Sixth sense *Victoria Gawne*	51
Paramedicine at sea *Niall Carty*	53
Some people see *Kirsty Wood*	55

Zero to one hundred *Anonymous*	57
Finding the essence of being a paramedic *Nich Woolf*	58
Butterflies *Craig Lusk*	61
A tipsy mess *Emma Jane Briggs*	62
Privilege *Anonymous*	63
All is fine *Scott Hardy*	64

Night Shift

The night shift *Karen Scott*	66
Click *Kaitee Robinson*	67
Unconditional *Natalie Sallis*	70
Eighteen minutes *Abigail Tucker*	71
What they don't teach you *Will Broughton*	74
A story of three parts: the elephant on the road *Wasim Ahmed*	75
COVID – the fight as a paramedic *Adrian McGrath*	78
Call me superstitious *Anonymous*	80
A community of hands working together *Adrian McGrath*	81

Connections 　*Carrie Ingram*	86
Time heals 　*Jen Jackson*	89
Heart sink 　*Andy McKinlay*	91
Echoes of loss 　*Matthew Herbert*	94
Perfectly formed yet incredibly tiny 　*James Grant*	95
Stress 　*Anonymous*	97
Waiting 　*Louise Sopher*	98
Christmas gifts 　*Monica Thompson*	99
Christmas in the ambulance service 　*Monica Thompson*	99
Critical Care 　*Monica Thompson*	99
My first year 　*Henry Thomas-Foy*	100
Not just a driver 　*Nicola Bromell-Pitter*	102
A bit of a high... 　*Steve Johnson*	103
Iron in the air 　*Emma Jane Briggs*	106
Camaraderie 　*Georgette Eaton*	110
The shifts roll together 　*Louise Sopher*	111

That time we stumbled upon a stabbing *Lucy McKenzie*	116
itsokaynottobeokay *Nic Haywood*	121
Heather *Anonymous*	123
The break of day *Charley Beale*	125
A guide for navigating the profession *Adrian McGrath*	129
Endnotes	131

FOREWORD

I was never one of those kids who knew what they wanted to be when they grew up. As a teenager, I did well in my GCSEs, but I failed all of my A Levels. It's a long back story, but I eventually ended up working in law, after returning to college aged 21, and then going on to do a law degree whilst working full time. However, in the recession of 2009, I was made redundant from the legal assistant job I'd finally made it into.

Whilst looking for a new job, someone recommended looking into the NHS – with a strong background in legal secretarial work, it was suggested I would find a good admin job with them. I went straight on to the NHS Jobs website and saw an advertisement for a student paramedic with the Yorkshire Ambulance Service. I thought *that sounds different*, I applied, and the rest is history!

I started my new role in January 2010. After an intensive initial few weeks of training, I was sent out on my first observer shift with an ambulance crew. I was obviously nervous, but the main thing that was playing on my mind was how I was going to react when I saw my first dead body, something I'd only ever seen on TV. It wasn't long before we got despatched to what we call a DOA (dead on arrival), but it didn't affect me in any of the ways I thought it would. Of course, I found the circumstances of the person's death tragic, and I can still picture the scene of that incident over 14 years later, but I would soon come to learn that often the hardest part of my job was the emotional side.

The role of a paramedic involves every circumstance you can ever imagine – from births to deaths, and everything in between. We sometimes refer to ourselves as a 'jack of all trades'. To our patients, we become what they need in what can be, at times, the direst of circumstances. As well as providing potentially life-saving treatment to those in their hour of absolute need, we consider the needs of their partners, their family, their carers.

I achieved a promotion to Clinical Supervisor in 2019, a role which involved working on a cardiac arrest response car. Little did I know that, less than a year later, the COVID-19 pandemic would hit and the following eight months or so would become the most difficult of my career. We could no longer take relatives to hospital with their loved ones, and sometimes I would know that it was potentially the last time they would ever see them. What we dealt with then will stay with me for the rest of my life.

This breath-taking anthology of paramedic stories made me both laugh and cry. Over my (almost) 15-year career, I have been in pretty much every one of the scenarios you are about to read. I view my job as such a privilege – to be the person who can not only help to save a life, but also help to change a life; to be the person who helps bring a new life into the world, and on a different day, the person who has the honour of holding an elderly person's hand whilst they take their last breaths. Although almost every shift has its challenges, it's also one of the most rewarding jobs in the world.

In 2009, finding out I was being made redundant felt like the worst thing that could possibly happen and I was nervous for my future – looking back, I now consider it one of the best things that ever happened to me. The pride, the sorrow, the joy and every other emotion which comes with our profession are described throughout the pages of this book which celebrates all that it is to be a paramedic.

Jules Swain
The Reading Paramedic
X: @thereadingpara
Instagram: @thereadingpara
TikTok: @thereadingparamedic

PREFACE

Across the country, at any given time, a paramedic will be boiling the kettle in their ambulance station crew room, their sanctuary between calls. These increasingly rare moments of respite are precious, offering a brief escape from the relentless pace of their work. As the tea steeps or the coffee brews, the crew room hums with the buzz of shared stories from recent shifts and past incidents, a space where camaraderie thrives amidst the tales of the extraordinary and the mundane. Here, laughter and reflection blend, providing solace and a momentary reprieve before the next call. The stories shared are not just about the job; they are about the people who do it, their resilience, their fears, and their triumphs.

Welcome to *Sirens and Stories*, the first anthology to capture some of these crew-room stories, penned by paramedics and ambulance staff from across the UK. Through these narratives, we aim to share the true essence of our profession, providing an insight into the challenges and rewards that define paramedicine. To do so, we must warn you of the content: this anthology includes accounts of traumatic events, medical emergencies, and other potentially distressing situations. Some readers may find the content emotionally challenging. We advise those sensitive to such topics to proceed with caution.

In this collection of stories and poetry, you'll encounter the humour that lightens our work and the deep, often sorrowful, reflections of those profoundly affected by their experiences. We believe it is crucial to support the continuous efforts of paramedics and their colleagues in ambulance services. Therefore, a percentage of the profits from this book will benefit The Ambulance Staff Charity (TASC). TASC is the only UK charity dedicated to supporting the mental health, physical rehabilitation, and financial wellbeing of the UK's ambulance staff, their families, students, and volunteers.

Like any profession, paramedicine has its own set of medical terms, acronyms and colloquialisms that form the foundation of our professional language. To help you navigate these terms when they appear in the narrative, we have implemented a numerical signposting system that directs you to a glossary at the end of the book.

There is no job in the world more rewarding than being the person called upon to help humanity on their worst day, stepping into the unknown and facing challenges in the knowledge that you can make an immediate and lasting impact on someone's life. We invite you to join us in our crew room, to share in our experiences as we provide an insight into the vital role paramedics play in the fabric of healthcare and society.

Georgette Eaton
Editor

DAY SHIFT

Provided that

If you can keep your head when all about you
are losing theirs and blaming 111.
If you can trust yourself when all others doubt you,
and refer them back, from where they've come.
If you can stoically wait and not tire from waiting
    (to handover),
or being DATIXed[1], or unjustly complained about.
Or being late off, don't give way to hating (and moreover),
stay true to yourself, and professional throughout.

If you can drive – and not let traffic cause frustration;
if you can finish on time – and not make that your aim.
If you can meet with ROLE[2] and return of spontaneous
    circulation,[3]
and treat those two impostors just the same.
If you can bear to hear the history you've taken,
twisted by patients who make you look a clown,
or watch the person you thought was broken
spring out of bed, as matron frowns;

If you can justify your best decision,
prepared to humbly get it wrong.
If you can teach yourself without derision,
and accept your weaknesses can make you strong.
If you can find yourself in the darkness of sorrow,
and provide the light by which others can see;
and give of yourself when there's nothing left to borrow,
except your will to respond when they call out: "help me!"

If you can talk in crew rooms, and keep your virtue,
or lead and still retain the common touch,
if neither Maccies nor missed meal breaks can hurt you,
and you can revel in the chaos – and enjoy it – but not too much.
If you can fill the tired hours of those unforgiving nights,
with the hope and redemption of the newly breaking sun,
you'll be ready for the world and all its tragicomic sights,
you'll be a great paramedic – job done.

Lawrence Hill
Associate Professor in Paramedic Science Education

The lament of a student paramedic

I wake up to another day,
and hear the sirens on their way.
I know that I have to be strong,
that I cannot get it wrong.

I've seen the worst that life can bring,
I've seen the pain that people cling
to every day, with every breath,
and every night, with every death.

And though I try to keep my cool,
I keep my feelings in a pool.
I can't help but feel the weight
of every life that's lost to fate.

It's hard to think of friends out having fun,
and I'm the one out on the run.
But I know that I have to be brave,
And that I have lives to save.

I feel the weight of every call
and know that I can't let it fall,
but for every life that we save,
another soul is sent to the grave.

I think about the road ahead,
and all the things that I have said.
I know that I have to be true,
and that I have to see it through.

I see the beauty in each day,
and in the work that comes my way.
So I know that I must play my part,
and that it's worth it, in my heart.

Carrie Martin
Student Paramedic
Ambulance Services

Welcome to the ambulance service

Despite it being well over seven years ago, one of the first incidents I attended as a student paramedic still sticks with me.

I was very excited to be in the ambulance. I had polished my shoes, ironed my uniform, and had everything ready in preparation for my very first day on placement. When I arrived at the station I was introduced to the crew and we made the vehicle ready. It wasn't long after that we were dispatched to a category 2[4] call, chest pain in an older man. On the way, I leant through the hatch between the back of the ambulance and the crew at the front, listening to the attendant (sat in the passenger's seat) as they explained what could potentially be happening, which assessments and possibly what treatment would be needed. As a first-year student I was nervous – the weight of my new role heavy on my shoulders – and keen to learn. Whilst we were on our way, the call was upgraded to a category 1[5] call, and control let us know that instructions were being given for bystanders to provide chest compressions. I felt the surge of speed, as the driver increased the pressure of their right foot on the accelerator. The attendant shouted a new set of instructions through, explaining which equipment we'd need to take into the job with us. Prior to the placement, my university programme had ensured we'd all completed a basic life support course, and I mentally prepared myself that I would be undertaking chest compressions in a few short minutes.

Arriving at the scene, we grabbed the equipment between the three of us, and I followed my crewmates up the garden path to the ground floor flat. The front door was locked. My crewmate frowned as he knocked urgently – I knew that callers were usually asked to open the doors to enable us to gain access to the patient without delay. A voice from inside shouted out a four-digit number for a keysafe to the right. Scrambling with the code, and then the keys in the door, we followed the sound of instructions being given out by one of our control room colleagues on the phone. It occurred to me that this bystander may have been undertaking chest compressions for some time by now, and I was keen to take over. We had bundled through the door of the living room together, when the attendant stopped abruptly and it was all I could do not to walk into the back of them.

A man was sat in a reclining chair, his bandaged legs raised, waving at us frantically to come into the room. "The ambulance is here now," he spoke into the phone before hanging up and dropping it onto the table beside his chair. A strong smell of urine and unwashed body assaulted my nose. A hospital bed was in one corner of the room, yellowed bedsheets pulled back.

"Where's the patient?"

He smiled up at us from the chair, "I've dropped the TV remote, pass it to me". Resting on the floor between the table and his chair was a remote so well used that it no longer had symbols on the buttons.

Back in the ambulance, the crew turned to me and said, "Welcome to the ambulance service!". Whilst this was the first time I experienced this, it certainly wasn't the last. Over time, I've learned that finding the humour in these situations is essential to staying sane amidst the chaos of emergency response.

Sarah Hennessy
Paramedic
Ambulance Services

Rats of the sky

We were once called to a man who had been trimming his tree with an angle grinder.

Not questioning his unconventional gardening technique, we met him holding a checked tea towel turned crimson to his hand in his front garden.

The makeshift bandage had managed to slow the bleeding somewhat, though unwrapping it revealed the bloody stump of his fourth finger.

Leaving my colleague to apply a new bandage and discuss options for pain relief, I headed to the angle grinder discarded at the base of the tree to try to retrieve the severed finger. With the incident occurring less than twenty minutes previously, my thoughts were that we may be able to provide the surgeons at the hospital with a good window of opportunity to reattach the digit.

Finding nothing amongst the foliage, my attention was drawn to a spray of blood on the greenhouse windows. Tracking the blood with my eyes, I saw the severed finger resting on the glass roof. Retrieving a nearby step ladder, I had just positioned it against the side of the green house when a flap of wings and rush of air startled me. I ducked instinctively, I looked around me to see a seagull flying away, the finger clenched firmly in its beak.

I returned to the patient and my crewmate, "About your finger..."

Richard Green
Senior Lecturer in Paramedicine
Education

You did your job

In my 15-year career, I've only truly saved one life. He'd collapsed in his living room, clutching his chest. His wife had called 999, and I was only a road away as a solo responder. Straight in, defibrillator pads on, shocked ventricular fibrillation.[6] I started chest compressions, the familiar feel of the pop of the sternum beneath my hands, as the ambulance crew walked in. Two minutes later, at the next rhythm check, he had a pulse. In the ambulance, his electrocardiogram[7] showed a myocardial infarction.[8] His consciousness was increasing all the time as we conveyed him to the cardiac department for PCI.[9] I doubt the consultant cardiologist would have believed my account had it not been for the recorded evidence from the defibrillator.

I happened to go back to the hospital at a later point in my shift, and I took the opportunity to follow up on the patient's progress. His wife welled up with tears as I entered the bay on the cardiac ward, closing the curtain behind me. She enveloped me in a tight embrace. He sat on the hospital bed, observing our interaction. I recounted the events to him, emphasising his fortunate outcome, and wished him a swift recovery. I lingered, anticipating that his response may include an expression of thanks. "You did your job," he said.

Anonymous

Are you the ambulance driver?[10]

I'm not just a driver
I attended your wife,
performed CPR
and saved her life.

I find out your history
I cannulate[11] too,
give drugs for your pain
to get you through.

I'm not just a driver,
you may ask me why,
I walked through the door
and smelt UTI.[12]

I read ECGs[7]
I auscultate[13] chests;
hairy ones, sweaty ones
and navigate breasts.

I'm not just a driver
I work as a team,
paperwork, observations
and keep the truck clean.

Replacing the bedding
I do other tasks too:
I clean up blood,
urine, vomit, and poo.

I'm not just a driver
My knowledge is vast,
just don't ask me which job
I have been to last...

At the "end of life"
I know my drugs.
When things get emotional,
I give great hugs.

I'm not just a driver;
the list goes on,
delivering babies
(though, to date, only one).

I worked throughout COVID and I'm a survivor,
I'm not just an average
ambulance driver!

Emma Chetwood
Paramedic
Ambulance Services

Biceps blues: a shower saga

We signed on for the start of our shift at 10am. We were immediately given a category 3[14] call: fell in shower, cut arm. The patient was a 40-something-year-old. Reading the notes, our eyes rolled: why does a man in his 40s need an ambulance because he's fallen in the shower and cut his arm?

We trundled the two miles into the town centre and saw three big, burly blokes waving us down outside a pub. Pulling up next to them, we saw one of them holding a blood-soaked towel to his upper arm.

Inviting him into the back of the ambulance, we ascertained he'd slipped in the hotel shower, his arm catching on one of the antique taps as he fell. He furrowed his brow as I chuckled at his remark about leaving half of his arm on the taps. He was broad shouldered, with a belly to match, and would have fallen hard and heavy. I unravelled the towel as I chatted to him, not expecting a spurt of blood to narrowly miss my head. I quickly covered it back up and held firmly to where I thought the bleeding had come from – the crook of his elbow, where the brachial artery lies. My crewmate applied the blood pressure cuff and pulse monitor to his other arm, setting the machine for automatic readings, and looked at me quizzically when I asked them to pass me the major trauma dressings bag. Now I was applying direct pressure, I could see the blood rising in the towel around my gloved hands. The first blood pressure was lower than I would have expected, his heart rate slightly higher than normal. My crewmate set about securing vascular access.

Gingerly peeling the towel back and shifting my fingers to apply some indirect pressure above where I thought the blood had come from, we saw the wound for the first time. A gaping hole was where his biceps should have been, the cavity filling quickly with the bright red blood of the arteries. I realised he hadn't been lying about leaving half his arm in the shower. We wasted no more time in applying a tourniquet[15] and administered a medicine (tranexamic acid) that would help his blood to clot.

One pre-alert to the nearest emergency department and a blue-light drive across town later, I handed over to the emergency medicine consultant in a resuscitation bay. The patient's blood pressure and pulse rate had markedly improved, and the exasperated consultant challenged us regarding our triad of treatment, which he predicted would be excessive for the injury sustained.

The consultant instructed a nurse to unravel the bandage whilst he began to loosen the tourniquet. A red arc of blood erupted, flooding down the patient's arm and the hospital trolley bed before pooling on the floor. He fumbled as he tightened the tourniquet, avoiding eye contact with me but having the decency to look a little abashed at the realisation that our treatment was, in fact, needed. Priceless.

Ashley Lucas
Paramedic
Ambulance Services

A nose for trouble

Some police constabularies employ their healthcare staff directly, to provide medical cover for detainees in custody, as well as medical services for police staff and other duties including taking and presenting forensic samples for prosecution. Paramedics are able to take on these roles, becoming a forensic healthcare professional (FHP) and undertaking additional, specialist, in-house training.

In my role as an FHP, I provided medical cover for two police custody units, several miles apart. One was a major crime centre, always busy, always demanding. The other was a rural town custody unit, half the number of cells but with some unique qualities that required a special sort of consideration, such as a prevalent and unpredictable recreational drug use that crossed all social groups.

It was always a risk leaving the big major crimes custody unit just in case you missed a new case coming in, or a current case took a new turn. But the smaller more rural custody unit needed visiting and had its own concerns. Because they do not have a full-time FHP and rely on sharing cover with the major crime centre, staff there often felt more vulnerable. They had suffered a death in custody not long before I joined the team, and it had been noted that some of the custody staff were subsequently, understandably, prone to anxiety over detainees' health. They often called for an FHP, outside mandatory responsibilities, and we often had to weigh up whether their concerns were worth the risk of leaving the detainees within the major crime unit.

One day a custody officer from the rural station called me. I knew him well. He was a very caring and diligent person, a keen first aider and an excellent custody officer. "I know that you're going to think I'm stupid but...," he started. I was in the middle of a busy day. That morning, all six FHPs on duty at several separate custody units across the county had processed a group of detainees accused of gang rape, taking DNA samples and juggling detainees to avoid any potential for cross-contamination.

On top of that, I had several detainees admitted to the major crime unit with medications and chronic concerns that had to be documented and organised to maintain their recommended care regime. I didn't want to leave my station, or break my flow, but I encouraged him to continue: "What have you got?"

"Well, we've got a woman in the holding cell waiting to be booked in and there's something not quite right about her." "What do you mean?" I asked. Something about the tone of his voice made me listen. "Well, as I say, you're going to say I'm being stupid, but she's only been here fifteen minutes and she's asked for two hot chocolates already."

It sounds silly, doesn't it? But I know this guy and I can hear that he's concerned in a slightly different way. I can hear that he's *sensed something* that he can't explain. They have limited first aid training, no medical equipment to check physiological observations such as blood sugar or blood pressure, and a limited ability to assess an acutely unwell patient. But they do have great instincts.

I asked a few quick questions: what's her colour like? What's her speech like? What's she doing right now? How is her demeanour? Is her breathing normal? Can you get a pulse rate? The answers to everything I asked came back positive. "I know it sounds silly, it's just as I say, there's something not quite right..." he said.

I'd already gathered the keys for the unmarked police car reserved for FHPs and scooped up my kit bag. I was thinking that, if nothing else, I could help them by offering support, making them feel protected, especially after the awful experience of managing a death in custody on their own when the FHP was remote. "I'm on my way," I said, "if anything changes and you are concerned, don't wait for me, call an ambulance." His relief was palpable, even over the phone.

It takes an average of 30 minutes to drive from one custody unit to the other. I knew instinctively there was something about this call, and it was all I could do to drive at normal road speed.

As I entered the custody unit I could sense immediately a change in atmosphere. I was met with "Oh, thank God you came," and was led immediately to a cell.

In the time between the custody officer calling me and my arrival, the detainee had been booked into custody, searched, and settled into her cell to rest and await interview. She had been chatty, relaxed, compliant and had raised no concerns with the sergeant. The custody officer who had called me had gone back to check on her and found her unresponsive just minutes before I arrived.

"I just knew something was wrong," he said, as I started my primary survey. She was of small stature, slim, with long hair scraped back into a ponytail. Easing back her eyelids, I saw pinpoint pupils. Opiate overdose. She was deeply unconscious, with the start of life-threatening respiratory depression. I prepared to administer the opiate reversal drug, naloxone, which was a standard item in my response bag. We had caught the progression of the overdose in good time. This would be an easy state to turn around, but quite a different story if it had gone on any longer, unnoticed.

It is very hard to keep a close eye on people in custody. A lay person might think it's easy, but it's not. Detainees nearly always lie down and often sleep, with nothing else to do. Distinguishing between someone who is asleep and someone who is unconscious due to the sudden onset of a medical condition, based solely on a CCTV image or a small window in a cell door, is extremely challenging.

The detainee responded well to the reversal drug, and made a good recovery. We sat her up and she drank her third hot chocolate. She was a lively character, very polite, very funny. The custody officer and I sat either side of her, me completing the consultation and he supporting by supplying the fresh hot chocolate. We smiled at each other over the head of this hapless, kooky and, mercifully, alive lady.

It is important not to judge in custody. To do your job really well, you must concentrate on who you are, what your profession is and perform with 100% consistency. But it's not always easy to know when to trust someone's instincts. I trusted the custody officer because I knew he was great at his job, and I knew from working with him previously that he had a "nose" for trouble. I'm not being superstitious, I'm being practical. For someone like him, who has experienced a traumatic experience, watched someone in his care die whilst waiting for professional medical back-up, it's different. He now has an ability to see trouble coming, and that's a really good skill to have which must be protected – it's my job to support him when he needs it.

Sarah-Jane Niles
Paramedic Practitioner
Primary Care/Ambulance Services

Sprain

Varus?[16] Valgus?[17] Erm...
No, I'm a Gemini. But,
She twisted her knee

Sneeze-on

Warmer weather. Sun-
Shine and rain, cough sneeze sniffle
Hay fever season

Zombie chicken pox

What is this red rash?
You've got zombie chicken pox!
Shingles ain't no fun

Monica Thompson
Advanced Paramedic Practitioner (Urgent Care)
Ambulance Services

The unlikely asylum seekers

A regular address we used to attend was a hostel for asylum seekers. Before it opened, there were articles in local newspapers protesting that the rate of crime would surely rise in the area, that such a hostel would contribute to the rising unemployment in the area and that the local health infrastructure wouldn't be able to support an increase in the local population. I've always hated this narrative.

On this day, we were called there to attend a call that had been redirected to the ambulance service by 111: a 37-year-old female with dizziness.

We arrived and, as usual, it took a while to find a parking space on the crowded residential street. This was no surprise with it being so close to the city centre. We buzzed the secure door at the bottom for entry, walked in and discussed with the staff member sitting behind a barred reception. There was an open-plan communal area next to us, busy with lots of children around. We were directed upstairs to the patient's room. It always seemed loud here no matter the time of day: an infant crying, children running up and down hallways, adults speaking in raised voices. The corridors and carpets were tidy, if a little grubby – undoubtedly from the high volume of footfall they saw. As we walked up the stairs, I remembered a patient I had attended not too long ago in a small room with her husband and five children; they shared two single bunk beds and a thin mattress on the floor between them. I wondered if the set-up for this patient would be similar.

I heard the door unlock from the inside, and we were greeted by the patient's husband. He was immaculately groomed, dressed in a crisp tunic. His appearance, and that of the bare room which was well kept and tidy, seemed at odds with the noise and grubbiness in the corridor and the surrounding rooms. Behind him, our patient was lying on one of the two single beds, a cool flannel on her forehead. As we entered, she sat up, dislodging the flannel, and thanked us for coming. She explained her symptoms, her concerns, and I conducted a neurological examination. Concluding that a peripheral vertigo[18] was the only symptom, I called 111 to arrange a telephone call with a GP to discuss the most appropriate treatment. We made small talk while I was waiting for the call-back.

They were very unhappy with their current living situation, not least because of the noise. Many of the residents had recently become unwell with vomiting and diarrhoea, they suspect because of the poor hygiene standards of the kitchen staff. They had been living on fruit for the past two days, the only thing they trusted that wouldn't make them unwell again. Their £8 per week allowance did not stretch very far to making more nourishing meals. He told me he was a banker, but that his wife earned more than him in their home country as a scientist. They had lived in Dubai, no children, had a large house with an outdoor garden, and two Range Rovers.

"How did you end up here?"

They looked at each other, it was a look that seemed to say, "Should we?". She nodded at him, signalling her approval.

He sat on the bed to relay their story. He had lived in another country in the Middle East before moving for work and meeting his wife. Life was going exceptionally well. But then one day he was contacted by someone in a position of power from his home country. He was told that his compliance and discretion were mandatory. They wanted him to assist in their child trafficking operation. He was a banker with no criminal record and no connection to this world. He ignored the emails. He couldn't believe that it was real, and thought it must have been some sort of hoax. But they became more persistent, and progressively threatening. They started to call him. They would turn up at his home. It began to seem very real. As it escalated, he considered what to do. Looking at his wife again, he said they talked about it together. He could comply, in the hope that whatever he needed to do would be over quickly so that they could resume their normal lives, but how could he? Once he complied with this request, who's to say they wouldn't ask for more? Most of all, how could he live with himself being complicit in the abhorrent crime of child trafficking? They told him they would kill his wife, his friends, his entire family if he refused.

They did the only thing they could do. They packed up their belongings, gave their house and car keys to their friend, and flew to the UK. For a while they stayed in hotel rooms under pseudonyms. They withdrew their savings to live on until they could establish themselves and find work here; after all, they both have excellent qualifications. However, not too long after entering the UK, they found that their bank accounts were frozen and they could withdraw no more money. He speculated that maybe this was because they were missing from their home country, or maybe even it had been achieved by the group that were making the threats. With no money, no jobs, no fixed address, their only option was to seek asylum. And here they found themselves in a small room in a loud, busy hostel – in a city they had not heard of before entering the UK, desperate to find work and establish themselves here. One of the things they found the most difficult was their inability to continue in the careers they had enjoyed.

We were interrupted by a call-back from the GP. I briefly explained the patient's symptoms and offered her the phone for the GP to ask some clarifying questions. I sat, dumbfounded at what I had just heard. I looked down to see I had barely written any paperwork. My reverie was then again interrupted by my radio; control were asking for an estimated time to clear.

With a prescription and follow-up consultation arranged for the patient, we completed our paperwork and left. I don't know what became of them, but I hope they were successful in obtaining asylum – and that they could pick up their careers again. The local papers never capture the real reasons why individuals may seek asylum.

That's the thing with our role. It's not just our experiences and our stories, it's the stories of our patients that we carry with us, too.

Lucy McKenzie
Paramedic
Ambulance Services

Bedside intruders

When I first trained for the ambulance service 17 years ago, working in London, I thought that traumatic incidents were "where it is at". To be fair, the ambulance service was quite different then, and trauma made up a higher percentage of our workload. I enjoyed trauma training, took a special interest in trauma jobs, and I fully expected to specialise in critical care. However, several years later in a different ambulance service, in a rural community, the prevalence was of calls oriented towards primary care. I decided to bite the bullet and change my direction to specialise in primary and urgent care, and I applied to work in a rural general practice. What ensued was a fascinating insight into a world I barely appreciated – an experience I would compare to *All Creatures Great and Small*, but with humans. In my role I was employed to perform only the home visits. There were funny calls, sad calls, weird calls. Addresses I dreaded, addresses I looked forward to. I met some wonderful people and was honoured to be a part of our communities' lives, to guide a recovery or support a patient as they approached the end of their life. It was far more varied than I had expected.

One day, I had a home visit booked to an elderly lady who lived alone but was supported by her daughter. Her daughter answered my knock at the front door and invited me in. The lady was very arty and there were creative endeavours throughout the house as we made our way from the front door to the patient's bedroom. My patient lay in bed comfortably, well cared for, bright and healthy looking in colour, smiling as she greeted me – grateful for my visit. We shared a brief conversation about arts and crafts, revealing mutual interests. Her daughter joined our conversation, sitting at the end of the bed with an arts and craft magazine in her hand. I was so wrapped up in our conversation, I almost couldn't remember why I had been called until the patient had a coughing fit. Remembering she may have a suspected chest infection, I proceeded with a relaxed history take and examination.

I was poised over her, leaning in closely with my stethoscope placed to listen to her lung sounds, when something caught my eye. A flying ant. It crashed into the pillow next to her head. I was just about to say something about it and flick it away when quite suddenly the pillow exploded with black flying ants. Hundreds of them. Several were now on her forehead and running across her chest. I half fell backwards off the side of the bed. The daughter, who had been sitting peacefully chatting about some craft in her magazine, emitted a high-pitched scream as she jumped to her feet. The patient was staring back at us in confusion, only partially aware of the full extent of the flying ant situation. I was struggling to verbalise sounds of reassurance when the daughter rolled up the magazine and began swatting at the ants, including those crawling across her mother. The patient, now thoroughly alarmed, began to struggle, fending away the rolled-up magazine brandished by her daughter and trying to move away from the ants next to her head. Having regained some of my senses, I began to sweep the ants from the bed. Instinctively, they flew towards the daylight streaming through the window, which the daughter quickly opened. As the insects were vacating the bedroom, we caught each other's eye. Simultaneously aware of our predicament, we all started laughing. Literally tears of laughter. Working together, the daughter and I cleared the infestation and resettled the patient in the living room, so we could finish the assessment along with a much-needed cup of tea for all involved.

Together, we came up with a plan: I was to return to the practice and hand over my assessment findings to the duty GP, recommending a course of antibiotics. I left the house still chuckling to myself at the unprecedented ordeal I'd been a part of.

Back at the practice, I called in to chat with the GP, as was our routine. I delivered a short, sharp handover as was this particular GP's preference and then at the end mentioned the ants, laughing as I recalled the story. She looked back at me, initially confused, and then shrugged as she turned back to her notes to issue the prescription.

You can miss a lot by not visiting someone in their home. I reasoned that the experienced GP had probably been involved in a few ordeals herself, but unfortunately the demands of primary care now meant that it was simply more effective for her to be based at the practice. I couldn't help but feel a little sorry for her, that I could experience some of the best parts of primary care, out in the community I was part of.

Sarah-Jane Niles
Paramedic Practitioner
Primary Care/Ambulance Services

A job that took us by surprise

Under the bright midday sun, we were on standby next to the river that winds its way lazily through my city when our sunny reprise was interrupted by the radio. I was a student, working on the solo response car with my mentor.

> Category 4[19]
> 40-year-old male
> Call from police
> Self-harm – cuts to wrist

That someone could feel so low as to harm themselves seemed at such odds with the sunny weather. Between the sirens as my mentor drove to the call, we speculated that a relative or friend of the patient on scene had likely called the police and that, as it was a category 4 (low priority), the wounds were unlikely to be serious. This type of call was commonplace, and these were the usual findings, though the time of day would usually be late evening or the early hours of the morning – the hours of darkness seemed to be when some people felt at their lowest. I still find it difficult not to speculate on the way to a job.

We arrived at a modern small complex of flats in an affluent area of the city, the entrance given away by a police car outside and a police officer standing in the doorway of a ground floor flat. His face was grave. The curtains were drawn on the floor-to-ceiling windows either side of the door. As I entered, my mentor behind me, I clocked a large blood stain tracking up one of the beige curtains from the floor. The floor was covered with congealed pools of blood. We followed the police officer into a large open lounge space with a kitchenette on the far side and windows overlooking a shared communal space in the middle. There was a large, blood-stained kitchen knife on the otherwise tidy breakfast bar. My mentor was intercepted by another police officer. Half listening to their handover, my eyes traced a wide blood trail from the kitchen to a mirror, which then lead through the door to another hallway. The police officer beckoned me from the doorway, and I followed her and the trail of blood droplets to a bedroom.

The patient was sitting upright on the edge of the bed, alert. His eyes and mouth were wide open, he was grey, his expression one of shock. There was a large gaping wound to his throat, with what I can only describe as a congealed waterfall of dark red blood clinging to his neck, his t-shirt, and his trousers. I realised I could see his trachea. There were some other wounds to his wrists, slightly oozing blood, but nothing fast.

I called my mentor's name.

He entered and stopped in his tracks – his eyes wide as he took in the patient. I imagine I must have done the same as I entered a few seconds before.

Approaching the patient, I asked if I could place dressings on his wounds. He nodded gently. A fresh stream of blood trickled from his neck.

I opened the major trauma pack. My mentor shone a torch to illuminate the wound to his neck. His trachea appeared to be intact. My mentor asked if he could swallow, we saw his trachea move up and down. I could not help but feel a little fascinated by this – anatomy I am taught but which should remain hidden. My mentor got on the radio to ask for back-up – we were in a car and couldn't convey the patient. His breathing was quick, but he did not appear to be struggling. He was quiet and we encouraged him to lie back on the bed, keeping his head and neck elevated. He accepted an oxygen mask as I checked observations. Unsurprisingly, his blood pressure was low – though his breathing rate and oxygen saturations were stable.

The nearest crew were 40 minutes away. The critical care team was on another call and unavailable. The nearest BASICS doctor[20] was 25 miles away. In a time before regional trauma centres, we already knew that the nearest hospital (less than ten minutes up the road) was on divert to the next hospital a further ten miles away. My mentor asked for anything control could send. Answer negative, on the radio. We were shit out of luck.

We asked one of the police officers to retrieve some more bags from the car. Given the blood loss, and the patient's physiological observations, we needed to prepare for imminent cardiac arrest. After some cannulation attempts into veins made poor by hypovolaemia,[21] my mentor managed to insert a very small one. Not ideal, but better than nothing. This was before we carried trauma dressings or medicines that assisted in blood clotting. We just had basic bandages. We got some fluids running. We prepared airways, applied defibrillator pads, got everything ready in case our patient took a sudden turn for the worse. All the time, he was alert, fully conscious, quiet, and co-operative. His face passive and grey. It all felt very surreal. Not much changed, his blood pressure improved a little, we continued to monitor. Waiting.

I heard the sirens with relief. An ambulance crew arrived, a BASICS doctor hot on their heels. I relaxed just a little bit in that moment. We started to hand over: 40-year-old male. A neighbour saw blood on the curtains and called the police. The police arrived and requested an ambulance. We described how we found the patient, his observations and what we had done so far.

The doctor looked at the patient, then at the monitor, pondered, then said he would make some calls to figure out which hospital we could convey to. We prepared the patient to transfer onto the ambulance stretcher, reassessing him frequently as we moved him. He continued to be alert and quietly obliging to our requests. I wondered what must have been going through his mind. I thought about him making his wounds, walking around his flat, looking in the mirror, sitting on the bed and waiting. Just waiting.

The doctor entered the ambulance and updated us. He had made a call to the local hospital, which despite being "on divert" had accepted. The doctor said he didn't care if all they could offer us was a trolley, he already had a team – us.

We arrived and they had made a space in Resus. We handed over. My mentor started on the paperwork, I made us all a tea. We sat down and had a short debrief with the doctor. He was impressed by how calm we were – especially waiting just under an hour for further help to arrive. I felt aglow at the compliment. Overall, a job well managed. We went back to station to clean and restock; my mentor and I hosed down each other's boots of the congealed blood.

Sometime later, my mentor managed to follow up what happened. The patient went to theatre where the wound to his neck was surgically managed. There was damage to his jugular veins, but not carotid arteries or trachea – which would have undoubtedly led to a very different outcome. He was discharged from hospital only days later.

What I remember most about this job was the feeling of being stuck, just the two of us, waiting for it all to take a turn south, and the relief when back-up arrived. A decade on, I can still see the way his eyes looked so wide when I walked in, how quiet and willing he was to allow us to treat him. Even now, I feel a sadness for him.

Lucy McKenzie
Paramedic
Ambulance Services

Another life saved

Aged 21, I had been on the road as a newly qualified paramedic for just about a month, and this was my first serious call. I read the mobile data terminal:[22] difficulty breathing, anaphylaxis.

I knew the clinical practice guidelines for this, having practised what felt like a thousand times during my degree. Life-threatening emergencies like this are rigorously practised at university so that by the time we would be attending one, the treatment would be second nature. But that didn't stop the flutter of nerves as we drove to the job. No amount of scenario practice can capture the intensity of being the one responsible for the life in front of you.

This was my first real experience of that responsibility.

My colleague was driving, an emergency care assistant[23] (ECA), called Tom. We had established at the start of the shift that he had been in the ambulance service more years than I had been alive, and was old enough to be my grandfather. With a slightly stooped back, mop of grey hair and wispy beard, he had the stereotypical grandfatherly appearance. ECAs are exactly what their job titles imply, they assist the paramedic in the provision of emergency care. I was somewhat comforted to be attending my first real emergency with someone as experienced as Tom, but also wary that the clinical responsibility would still be all mine, as the registered clinician. Whilst happy to follow instructions from paramedics, Tom was not known on the ambulance station for his ability to pre-empt the requirements for emergency care like other ECAs.

It felt like we drove for an age. The job was out in the middle of nowhere, rural Berkshire. It was a cloudless, gorgeous blue-sky British summer's day, and driving through the tiny country lanes between fields and forests almost made you forget the fact that you were racing under blue lights to an emergency.

We arrived at the long drive from the road, which would take us to the location we were given. As we approached this big house we saw him, a middle-aged man sitting on his patio chair in front of the red-brick Victorian house. Surveying the area around the casualty for danger (to myself or them) is one of the first considerations in emergency care, and through the bifold doors to the kitchen I glimpsed a pot of tea and mug on the kitchen island. But he was alone, red and puffy. Sweating. Gasping for air. Panicked.

I knew from his appearance that we didn't have much time. I asked him if he thought he was having anaphylaxis. We wouldn't normally do this, normally we would ask the patient more details of what led them to this moment, but time was of the essence. He nodded, gesticulating to a white suit with a round hood and veil. I knew immediately: bees.

"Is the ambulance there now?"

I could hear the call-taker's voice coming from the mobile phone that sat open on the patio table. He didn't even have the strength to finish the phone call.

"We're here," Tom said, ending the call whilst he was setting up a mask attached to an oxygen cylinder. Good, he didn't need prompting from me. He knew the gravity of the situation.

The patient's hand was against his chest as he fought to breathe. Panic etched in every line on his face, in his eyes, as I started drawing up the drugs required to save his life. I knew that if we didn't do something soon, he'd go into cardiac arrest.

I worked automatically, those hours and hours of scenario training guiding my hands. Drawing up the first drug: adrenaline. 0.5 mg in 0.5 mL 1:1000 solution, and then administering it by intramuscular injection. Right arm. As I plunged the syringe, Tom was removing the patient's glasses to apply an oxygen nebuliser[24] mask, which was pushing through the second drug, a bronchodilator[25] called salbutamol. Salbutamol works by opening the air tubes in the lungs, and Tom was making it secure enough to ensure as much precious oxygen as possible would find its way into the patient's already narrowing airways.

Whilst the patient had already indicated it was a bee sting, both anaphylaxis and life-threatening asthma attacks present in the same way. I didn't have time to get all the details from the patient, he was too sick. Time was of the essence, so the initial phase of treatment covered both eventualities.

I talked as I worked, in what I hoped was a soothing pitter-patter of introducing myself and Tom, explaining what I was doing, and what the plan was to help him. The panic was still in his eyes. He was still gasping, his whole body heaving to try to get as much oxygen in as possible.

I moved to the next drug, though this would require me to gain intravenous access.[26] I had five minutes before the next dose of adrenaline, so I had time. But he was peripherally shut down. His body was shutting down. He was going to die. My hands trembled slightly as I advanced the needle through the skin at the crook of his elbow. He didn't even flinch. It felt like a tiny tube of metal had never been so important. I was aware Tom was flitting around, hooking the patient up to our monitoring screens. Vascular access gained, I glanced at the monitor, which Tom had positioned on the metal Victorian patio table against which the patient was sitting. His heart rate was alarmingly high, and his blood pressure alarmingly low. It seemed so odd to have such grave physiological observations against the backdrop of green fields and a clear blue sky.

I started the patient on fluids – large volumes of fluid may leak from the patient's circulation during an anaphylactic reaction, and the low blood pressure and fast heart rate were indications of shock. I hooked the 500 mL bag up on the trellis that screened part of the patio from the driveway. Ambulances don't come with portable drip stands, and Tom was far too useful to me to be standing limply holding a bag of fluid, waiting for it to run its course into the patient's body.

Five minutes was up. He was still gasping. I gave the next dose of adrenaline. This time, in the other arm. This wasn't deliberate, it was just the nearest to me, having switched my position whilst hanging up the fluids.

He began to improve. His breathing calmed, and my monitor showed his heart rate slowing – though it was still faster than normal. I could see the panic lines that had been etched around his eyes fade a little. He looked at me, his blue eyes teary.

"Thank you."

"I'm not finished yet," I told him.

At least I could finally ask his name, confirm he had been stung by a bee, and what time, now he could speak a few words at a time. However, he wasn't yet out of the reaction – his body was still in shock. The adrenaline hadn't worked on its own.

Next up was an antihistamine, chlorphenamine.[27] I turned off the fluids to give the medication by a slow injection in the access in his arm. More pitter-patter chatter as I worked, talking through what I was doing, asking questions about the patient. I needed as much information as I could get from him in case the allergic reaction overcame him again.

It was working. He was no longer heaving to breathe. But he wasn't back to normal. I could have given another adrenaline dose at this point, but I opted to continue the initial treatment regime and administer steroids. Hydrocortisone must be injected slowly intravenously, and our clinical practice guidelines at the time outlined that it may help prevent or shorten protracted reactions.

I weighed up the decision in less than a nanosecond: more adrenaline, but he was improving, or slow injection of steroids. If I started the steroids, I couldn't rush them. They must be administered slowly, or I would risk causing his blood pressure to plummet further. If I misjudged and he needed further adrenaline, it would delay the third dose – potentially missing the treatment window.

I went with steroids. He was improving all the time, speaking more words together, his vital signs improving. I continued my pitter-patter chatter, about the weather, about the flowers on the trellis. I wonder now what he must have thought of me, a young blonde girl chatting to him about the garden whilst he was experiencing one of the most life-threatening events anyone can.

But just like that, the pentad of drugs worked together. He really was improving. Tears flowed more freely down his cheek, bunching about the nebuliser[24] mask – which was now just administering oxygen – and flowing around the mask to his chin.

My brain began to switch back on. I remember hearing Tom.

"Right," he said. "Now what?"

It had all happened so quickly. He was improving. It was working.

This became its own strange issue. I didn't really know what to do. I'd followed the clinical practice guidelines, the protocol for anaphylaxis, and the treatment had worked. What now? He was getting better. That's not in the guidelines. The guidelines tell me what to do if it gets worse, which in this case would be resuscitation for cardiac arrest. I didn't know what to do as the patient got better.

He'd need to go to hospital. Allergic reactions are sneaky like that, and they can reoccur after a refractory period, as some of the drugs wear off. I knew we had to take him to hospital in case he had another reaction when the adrenaline wore off... but other than that I wasn't really prepared for things to go *well*.

It was all very surreal. I would soon learn that the word *normal* didn't exist in the ambulance service. The extreme and the mundane wrapped intimately around each other, each day unpredictable.

On this day, the hot sun contrasted against the scene that had just taken place. Our patient was moments away from dying on a day that would be one of the summer's best. Somewhat stabilised, though still hooked up to our monitoring equipment, fluids and oxygen, he initially protested as Tom moved the ambulance stretcher next to the seat on which he was sat. Aside from the whole nearly dying thing, he was going to miss the rest of the beautiful day he had planned to spend in the garden. Like, thank you for saving me but I feel so much better now, is it really necessary for me to go?

Yes. Yes it is.

We called in a pre-alert and raced back through the beautiful countryside. I don't remember what we talked about on the drive back to the hospital. Probably the weather, maybe the bees. Keeping up that general pitter-patter whilst I documented our treatment, reading the times I had scrawled on the back of my glove as I provided the treatment. Fifteen minutes. From the first dose of adrenaline to the final drug, the hydrocortisone. That was it, just 15 minutes in which we changed his life dramatically. He wasn't the only person with adrenaline coursing through his veins.

It wasn't long before we were at the emergency department. The emergency medicine consultant I handed over to frowned sceptically when I listed the drugs I had administered, looking at the patient who was sitting up on the stretcher in a significantly better condition than at my arrival to him less than an hour earlier. I wasn't sure whether I was relieved or not when the patient added he had indeed felt his death was imminent. This at least seemed to convince the doctor.

I met Tom outside, who had been busy cleaning down the stretcher and equipment, and restocking kit. And that was us, onto the next job. Another life saved.

Anonymous

Memories

I once attended a 999 call to a man who died in tragic circumstances. He was a young man, in his early thirties, and he fell off a ladder in his back garden. He was simply putting up a washing line and had slipped, hitting his head on the patio and sustaining a skull fracture. I remember the incident vividly because the man was so young, and he had fallen only the height of an average step ladder. His wife was heavily pregnant at the time. We did everything we could, but he was pronounced dead in the hospital.

Some 14 years later, I was called to a teenager who had sustained a minor injury in the town centre. Following assessment and treatment, she was well enough to go home and rest. I asked if anyone could pick her up. She told me that her mum would be at work and that her dad had died. As you do in these situations, I said I was so sorry to hear that and she shrugged, "I never knew him because he died before I was born."

"Oh no that's awful."

"Yes," she said, "It was for my mum. He fell off a ladder..."

She stopped as she saw my eyes widen in disbelief. I looked at her home address on my paperwork, memories flooding back as I made the connection.

"You went to my dad, didn't you?" Tears began pouring down her cheeks.

I was struck by emotion. We had a connection. A strange connection but a connection nonetheless.

She rang her mum and we arranged that we would drop her home.

The house had been updated with the times, but otherwise had changed very little. Her mum recognised me as I followed her daughter to the front door. She smiled wryly as she offered me a cup of tea, saying she hadn't had the chance to offer me one the last time I'd been in the house. I didn't know what to say to her. I told her that I had thought about them both now and again, when I'd driven down that street. She cried and thanked me. Despite the tragic outcome, she thanked me.

Some memories live with us forever.

Neil Armstrong
Paramedic
Ambulance Services

More than medicine

Since I was a newly qualified paramedic, I've been deeply passionate about palliative care. My experiences in facilitating calm, dignified, and pain-free deaths have fuelled my determination to ensure that more patients can have their end-of-life wishes honoured.

I now work in primary care, and my story is the legacy of a patient whom I was able to support in the last weeks of his life. He had terminal lung cancer and was discharged from hospital care to receive palliative care only. One Tuesday, I was tasked to visit him at home. Sitting with him and his wife in their living room, I noticed he was wearing a Harley Davidson t-shirt. As a keen motorbike rider myself, we got chatting and his face lit up when talking about his racing days and old bikes he used to own. One of my tasks of the visit that day was to discuss with him his wishes for his care at the end of his life – and how we, as a primary care team, could support him. He'd like a motorbike escort for his funeral – could I liaise with his family to provide that when the time came?

This wasn't the planning I had in mind, and I thought about his request over the coming days. He was so passionate about bikes, I thought; why wait until he is no longer with us to experience this? At our review the following week, I mentioned this to his wife. She thought it would be wonderful for him to "hear the roar of the engines" one last time – but how could we arrange for some bikes to come to the house? The biker community is close, and we reached out on social media to find local bikers who would be willing to meet and provide a ride past for the patient. At the request of his wife, we would keep it a surprise for him. Within 24 hours the post was shared 135 times.

On the day, 41 bikes and pillions joined me to surprise my patient. For a patient who had been in bed for two weeks, with decreasing quality of life and increasingly limited interactions outside his home, the roar of our engines brought him outside his house. Several bikers stopped, and he was able to revel in his memories and admire the bikes; he was once again part of a biking community. Tears were shed by the patient, his family, the bikers, and yes, even myself.

Some time later, I was part of the smaller escort for his funeral. The family expressed profound gratitude for the end-of-life memories that went beyond medication management, caregiving, and loss. The fulfilment I had from this kindness, the difference in moving beyond medicine to focus on the *person* at the end of their life, will remain etched in my memory for eternity.

Gemma Butler
Paramedic and Trainee Advanced Clinical Practitioner
Primary Care

Around the mess table

Slam the side door for an out-of-system break, running to the loo as over six hours is hard for the bladder to take.

Around the mess room table, the moaning, analysing, the top trumps, the "what would you do", the silence and flirting too; mate, you making a brew?

The microwave "ping" and the out-of-date milk. You sit on the chairs that are sometimes beds and you hear "warning this vehicle is reversing" too. The urn is always hot and ready for the returning crew. They walk through the door and hear a shout; Who'd like a brew?

Burning eyes, hysteric giggling, and the stillness of your body screaming at you. Yep, that's right it's 4 in the blinkin' morning. Caffeine, we depend on you.

Twisted banter, laughter, and dark humour too, therapy perhaps or deep-rooted trauma that no one sees within you. Tears, frustration, pain, sometimes despair, an arm around your shoulders, bonds so strong never broken. We are a different kind of soldier.

Another brew as the shift is ending, a slow drive home, you're so fatigued it seems never-ending. A quick snack and off to bed, blackout blinds down, and minimal sound.

The alarm goes off, wash, uniform boot, and back for another round. "Ting ting", spoon mixing the fresh milk from the last crew. Ah, nothing quite like that first-shift brew.

If the mess room table could talk, I wonder what it would say. I wonder whether it would care for us in some old-fashioned way. Would it guide us with wisdom and words about life or would it respond despairingly at how harsh we can be? We never take our own advice.

Or would it say nothing as it's a bloody table, of course!

Next time you are sitting around a mess table, maybe stop and think once or twice, what would it say if it were able? What if it weren't just a table?

Karen Scott
Lecturer and Simulation Lead for Paramedic Program
Education

Naji (Survivor)

As well as being a paramedic who works in two ambulance services in the UK, I also volunteer in humanitarian work. This story is from my time working on a humanitarian mission in Ukraine during the war.

In Ukraine I was the training lead for a German charity called Cadus. I was tasked with setting up a medical education project to help local charities working in frontline towns providing humanitarian aid or assisting in the evacuation of elderly and vulnerable people from these places to safer areas in the west of the country. To understand what these groups needed to learn, I decided to work alongside them. I thought that by assisting with their work I would be better able to create meaningful educational content tailored to their specific needs. This story is from when I was welcomed into a local group, Base UA, around September 2022.

As I was embedded in the group I was acting as the team paramedic whilst on missions. On this day, the team was going to a newly liberated village near the frontlines, which had seen some intense fighting very recently. The plan for the mission was to do a needs assessment to see how to best support the local population. This was a rather concerning mission as, although it was unlikely that we would experience any shelling (the frontline had moved far enough by this point), there was a high risk from UXOs[28] – particularly from butterfly mines.

Having worked in these frontline areas for a while by that point, I had started including dog and cat food as a part of my day-to-day kit. In these areas, many dogs and cats had been left behind by their owners as they fled their homes. I'd never thought of myself as a huge lover of animals, but it simply broke my heart to see them all scampering around visibly hungry; I thought the least I could do was give them some food when it was safe to do so.

So, on this mission I had gathered a large number of cats and dogs up to our van by feeding them, when I noticed a kitten which was limping, his bone visible on one of his back legs. This pitiful wee ginger kitten came right up to me and my colleague, pressing against us and vying for our attention. Seeing how injured he was, I had a discussion with the team leader and we decided that the right thing to do was to take him back to our base and speak to a vet, even if it meant just a few days of spoiling and providing him with as much food and cuddles as this little cutie's heart desired before he passed.

We put him in a cardboard box with some treats and brought him with us to base. Upon proper assessment of his leg, it became clear that this wasn't an open fracture but rather an infected wound which was not healing and had gone all the way down to the bone. So, with the use of some telehealth assessment from a vet, I got proper instructions on how to manage this wee chap until we could organise medevac to a bigger city to a vet who could properly manage this presentation; the base was in a small city about 20 km from the fighting and all the vets had left.

And that is how I found myself doing my first ever bit of veterinary medicine. Word of advice to other paramedics who might stumble into doing accidental veterinary care – kittens bite and scratch considerably more than our standard patients! Luckily, I soon realised this and so manoeuvred others into holding him whilst I washed his wound and changed his dressing – strangely these volunteers rarely agreed to help a second time. Also, since little kittens take little amounts of antibiotics, we faced the not-so-little challenge of administering to our patient one 20th of an antibiotic pill. Possibly not the most handsome bit of precision medicine, but the best we could manage in the circumstances.

After a few days of care in the base, the head of mission for the charity I was working with visited to check in and have some meetings. Little did he know he would have to medevac this darling wee kitten the six-hour drive back to Dnipro where Cadus were based. This guy is a total sweetheart, but being a major dog person and allergic to cats, it's fair to say he was not happy with me. Thankfully he's also enough of a softy to agree to this mission. And so, the kitten was given a brand-new box and a prime space in the front of our ambulance, and driven back to Dnipro – only using my boss's jumper as a toilet a few times on the way back.

The care of the kitten was then taken over by our medical volunteers.

He was given the name Naji by some Palestinian friends – Naji means survivor in Arabic, and this wee kitten is for sure a survivor. A very kind-hearted anaesthetist from Germany managed to get Naji appropriate papers and he was taken back to Munich for further care, including some very expensive surgery.

Naji is now living with a family just outside Munich and has a dog as a friend and a very loving family taking care of him.

Even after years of being a paramedic and working in some of the most hectic environments, witnessing all manner of weirdness and suffering, this is one of the moments in my career that will always stay with me. Rescuing Naji was both surreal and deeply touching. As paramedics, we have to be flexible and empathetic clinicians. I never thought that would mean taking orders from a vet over the phone in a country at war – but apparently that, too, can be a part of our job.

Iain Campbell
Paramedic
Ambulance Services and Humanitarian Aid

Stepping into advanced practice

I spent six years developing my skills as a paramedic within the ambulance service, becoming familiar with the role and what it incorporates, before I looked to gain more experience. Ambulance work is a role I continue to enjoy, having the variety of patients, the thrill of weaving through traffic to get to someone and to make a difference, as well as being able to use a wide range of knowledge and skills to work autonomously.

The time came, however, to look at career progression and I initially moved into an education role. However, I missed seeing patients – helping people was the crux of my job – so looked at what was available for me to progress clinically. It seems that the most common clinical progression route is into primary and urgent care, perhaps as there's so much crossover from patients seen in the ambulance service into this setting. But for me, I felt a pull towards dealing with those who were critically ill or injured. I responded to a job advert for a training post as an advanced critical care practitioner and, admittedly to my surprise, was successful in getting the role.

My first day quickly arrived and as I stepped on to the critical care unit for the first time, I became acutely aware that I had never worked in a hospital before. The bustling tempo of the unit along with the variety of machinery humming along, emitting the odd alarm, was overwhelming. I was an unfamiliar face on a unit where everyone was busy. I had been given the name of someone to look for on my first day and so spent my first moments looking at people's name badges to find them. I was greeted with a smile, kindness, and the reassurance I'd be looked after – which was a relief. And so began the rapid, steep learning curve on my way to becoming an advanced critical care practitioner.

When you are used to working out of hospital, it is hugely different working in a hospital, which became apparent very quickly. Even things I thought I was good at became challenging, like conducting a physical assessment; I'd never listened to the lungs of a ventilated patient before, or assessed the haemodynamics[29] of a patient who had just had an aortic dissection repair. Paperwork, which seemed so simple in the ambulance service, became a nightmare, having to learn how to use a new system as well as learn about all the new acronyms and additional information that was now at my disposal as well. Then there was the daunting realisation that whilst I thought I was a good paramedic and enjoyed reading about a wide variety of clinical subjects, there were actually a huge number of things I didn't know existed. This transition of practice was complicated further by many of my colleagues assuming I came from a critical care nursing background where the scope of practice and skills is different to that of a paramedic. As such there were many times when I was asked to do something simple, like collect blood samples or place a nasogastric tube,[30] when I had never done this before. The patience and understanding of my consultant and nursing colleagues shone through in the moments where they would then take the time to teach me these skills.

Over time, things became easier, and my knowledge has developed alongside the additional skills required for the role. A year into my training I have achieved a huge amount, where I am now able to contribute more fully to the management of many of the patients on the unit. There is still much (much, much, much) more to learn and accomplish, but looking back at where I started, it is easy to see how much I have transitioned into this role and integrated into the team.

A typical day for me now would start with the morning handover round, where as a team we discuss what has happened overnight and if there are any specific issues that need addressing. Next, I review my patients, examining them holistically, interpreting various test results such as blood test or chest x-rays, before physically examining them and determining the next step for their treatment or rehabilitation. The level of knowledge required for this is huge, especially as every patient is different and will need a different care plan. This usually prompts some learning opportunities where I can discuss various conditions or treatment methods with my colleagues. Plans are then made during the main ward round with the consultants, which I am responsible for actioning for my patients under my delegation. I also seek opportunities with others on the unit as well, so if someone else's patient needs a new central line,[31] for example, I will add that to my list. This keeps me busy and makes the shift go quickly. I always come home tired, but equally I always come home having learned or achieved something new.

Jared Gooch
Trainee Advanced Critical Care Practitioner
Secondary Care

My father's legacy

It was the summer of 2008. I was in my late twenties and working as a supply chain analyst for a shipping company in Felixstowe, where I had worked for the last seven years. I had neither love nor hate for my job, and was content at my desk when I received a call from my dad that changed my life.

He had cancer. My world stopped and an immense void opened in both my head and my heart. Will he die...? What can I do...? What should I do...? My perspective on life changed.

It was not long afterwards that an advertisement in the local job section caught my eye: East of England Ambulance Service was recruiting student paramedics. I couldn't save my father, but maybe I could help someone else.

Sadly, I lost my dad in December 2018. He didn't see me graduate from my Master's degree or qualify as an advanced paramedic. But he did see me achieve my goal of registering as a paramedic, and I had the honour of supporting him as his disease progressed.

My passion as a paramedic has been supporting patients who receive palliative care at the end of their life. When I started as a student, many patients who called 999 for support in managing their symptoms at the end of their life would be taken to hospital – often their final journey. Now, as an advanced paramedic, I have the privilege of leading a project within my ambulance trust that supports advanced practice clinicians to provide symptom management to patients at the end of life within the community – allowing them to have a dignified and peaceful death in their preferred place of care.

Nick Williams
Advanced Paramedic (Urgent Care)
Ambulance Services

Not the rollercoaster you thought

Our days are up and down, not because we're running from saving one life to another, but because of the cycle of those automatic reactions to an incident: excitement? Frustration? Fear? Anxiety? Nothing?

Then arriving on scene where things will definitely change because the reality of the whole scene can never be on the incident notes. The shift in mindset from what you thought you were going to, to what you're now faced with.

Guilt from knowing what a patient needs but not having the resources to provide it, so you have to go for plan B.

The crewmate you haven't seen for ages and are keen to catch up with.

The one it's a real effort to get on with.

The one you're desperate to protect from certain things because you know they have their own worries on their mind.

The ones that are new, who you're not comfortable sharing how you're really feeling with yet, because you want to welcome them and support them settling in.

The one that knows your off days and doesn't let you forget they care.

The patients that really need you but "didn't want to bother anyone".

The ones that could be cared for at home if they had someone, anyone, for support.

The ones who play the system and who you have to do your best to be kind and professional with despite your own thoughts.

The ones whose ability to cope you can restore in unexpected ways.

The category 1[5] broadcasts and back-up requests while you're holding outside hospital, knowing you've been in that position yourself and remembering how it feels.

The inevitability of a late finish when you've planned something for yourself after work, for once.

The oncoming crew that helps you clean and restock, then makes you a cup of tea because you look like you don't even remember your own name any more.

This is ambulance work. We all feel it, whether we share it or not. Even if you're burned out and think you're not feeling much at all. We are the human element that operates a resource. We are not robots. To some it might be just a job, to others it's the only thing they could ever see themselves doing.

It's starting to sound clichéd with the "frontline hero" and the "system is broken" talk. So, let's focus on us now. We are a team. We are tired. But, if we acknowledge it and support each other, we can still learn and develop, and remember why we started.

You've got this. We've got this.

Anonymous

Intuition

I was in the final stages of studying for my Master's degree, whilst also working as a community paramedic rotating in primary care, and attending 999 calls in a rural area of Northern Ireland. My father was in hospital, in the intensive care unit, seriously unwell with a poor prognosis.

It was New Year's Eve. Primary care was hectic but jovial in atmosphere as everyone worked together to get last-minute appointments and late prescriptions sorted before the year's end and impending celebrations.

Then, a panicked phone call. A husband who was short of breath. Vague details. Panic... pain. I happened to overhear part of the conversation as I passed reception. Intuition? Opportunity? Something made me take the phone from the receptionist. Country people don't ring 999, they ring their GP. "Please help." I told her I'd be right out, informing ambulance control that I had picked up an emergency call and would need an ambulance to back me up. The voice, the panic... Something wasn't right. I never underestimate my role – doing the small things well and the big things better. I listen to my intuition.

In the living room, the patient was flat on the floor. I had a sense of impending doom. Process took over. Gave reassurance. Practicalities took over. Physiological observations, 12-lead ECG,[7] analgesia.[32] I could hear his wife on the phone to their daughter. This was someone's dad. My dad was dying in hospital. I had to save someone's dad, especially if I couldn't save my own.

The ambulance crew arrived. He went into cardiac arrest. Room cleared... successful defibrillation... we go again... reprieve. Still no ST elevation.[33] Decisions to be made. Nearest suitable hospital or cardiac centre for PCI.[9] Decision was easy. PCI... the history prior to collapse was distinctly cardiac. I left him in the safe hands of the ambulance crew. I stayed behind, alone in the room. His family had arrived by now, arms around their mother. All were in shock, not really considering the possibilities, just existing in the moment. We talked, I urged hope, prayer if appropriate. They shared stories of their husband, their father.

Now this is where I explain why I chose this particular story. We have incidents like this routinely, but I wanted to offer an account from the perspective of a community, from a responder, from a family. Response times have always been reportable, holding services to account, but rarely do we measure outcomes from a personal perspective. Rural communities have a unique footprint, a sense of altruism. You can't escape. The knock-on effect is immeasurable. Humanity, connection, empathy – all hallmarks of healthcare, but sometimes lost in the acute phase of illness. I reflected on my personal situation and the helplessness I felt with my dad's illness.

Regardless of one's belief in a higher power, the events of that day led to the salvation of more than one person. Seventy-two hours later, I visited the patient in the hospital and embraced his wife. She appeared different – happier, more at ease. They were making plans to relocate closer to their children, a second chance to spend their later years with loved ones. If circumstances had unfolded differently – if they had called just one hour later, if I hadn't been there as a community paramedic, if an ambulance hadn't been available – all these variables could have altered the course of a family's life in an instant. But somehow, they all worked in his favour.

As they did for my own family. My dad is still alive ... perhaps because someone else listened to their intuition to look after him, too.

Caroline French
Community Paramedic and Advanced Paramedic Practitioner
Primary Care

Keeping in touch

It was the late noughties, and we were called to a 60-year-old male having a stroke. On our way there, it was updated to cardiac arrest.

The family had been doing chest compressions for only nine minutes when we arrived. Four shocks[53] later, he had a return of spontaneous circulation[3] and respirations to boot. He regained consciousness on the way to the hospital.

The following week, we received a surprising update from the patient and his family. He had made a remarkable recovery and had been discharged from the hospital. They expressed immense gratitude for the care we'd provided – our quick response, recognition and treatment had changed the course of his life. Over the subsequent years, we maintained regular contact with them. We were honoured to attend his wedding, where he finally tied the knot with his long-term partner, and to witness the joy of seeing him walk his daughter down the aisle. We were also kept informed of his pride in his numerous grandchildren.

Almost 20 years later, I attended their funerals – both he and his wife succumbed to the virus during the pandemic. His daughter still keeps in touch, forever thankful for the two extra decades she had with her father.

Charlie McCourt
Clinical Support Officer (Paramedic)
Ambulance Services

Sixth sense

On entering the bedroom, it was apparent that the 24 hours of vomiting experienced by this 16-year-old was not caused by a seasonal bug. Worry was etched across both parents' faces as the young girl struggled to articulate her symptoms. We were thorough, systematic. Her physiological observations were normal, but she just *didn't look well*. I had this internal sense that something wasn't right, but we couldn't put our finger quite on the diagnosis to offer immediate treatment. And this was part of our decision to convey her to the hospital,

In the back of the ambulance, I went back over the history and progression of her symptoms. In my mind's eye, the clinical pieces fell into place: I couldn't rule out meningitis, a disease we don't often see, but which we are trained to recognise early and treat immediately. My sense that this was a serious matter stemmed from having that knowledge stored away, ready for moments like this very shift.

With the puzzle pieces falling into place in my mind, I relayed to our patient and her parents that, given the possibility of meningitis (her mother's eyes widened in horror at the mention of the word), I suggested we proceed with treatment. The potential harm from administering benzylpenicillin to a patient who didn't have the condition was far outweighed by the risk of not administering it to a patient who might. I acted fast, administering the medicine and making the paediatric emergency department aware of our impending arrival as my colleague drove us on blue lights to the hospital.

In hospital, a lumbar puncture confirmed meningitis. After a short stay in the paediatric intensive care unit, she was stepped down to a medical ward, and subsequently discharged home with no lasting effects. The consultant paediatrician I had handed over to at the hospital told me later that if I hadn't given benzylpenicillin when I did, at best she could have lost her legs – or worse.

In that instant, I came to understand the significance of those internal feelings of unease and the importance of trusting my gut instinct. As paramedics in emergency medicine, it's crucial to remain receptive and attentive to subtle cues, learning from them along the way. We often find ourselves piecing together a puzzle without always having a clear picture in sight. Thankfully, I've always been pretty good at jigsaw puzzles.

Victoria Gawne
Paramedic
Ambulance Services

Paramedicine at sea

It was the summer of 2017. I had volunteered to be deployed with the Irish Naval Service to the Mediterranean, off the coast of Libya, to rescue migrants who were attempting the perilous crossing from Libya to Europe. Every year, thousands of people were attempting to make this journey, resulting in large numbers drowning.

A typical rescue upon identification of boats in distress usually took upwards of six hours – from rescue, to triaging, and then processing. The boats they typically set out on usually have a maximum capacity of 30 people. However, these inflatables were dangerously overloaded, carrying 80–100 individuals on board. They had just enough fuel to reach 12–15 miles out from the coast into international waters. Typically, the distress call was initiated by the gangs on the shore, prompting a co-ordinated response from multiple agencies including those from Britain, Italy, Ireland, and Spain.

On several occasions, these overloaded boats capsized, resulting in many drownings. With a medical crew of four, consisting of paramedics and emergency medical technicians, and six first aiders, we had to deal with multiple drownings over a sustained period, with poor outcomes for most. A triaging system was implemented frequently due to the regular rescues encountered. Many of the migrants carried injuries including fractures, stabbings, burns – each with horrific stories of the treatment from their captors. Others would have uncontrolled medical conditions, such as diabetes, mental health problems, pregnancy-related issues, malnourishment, scabies – to name but a few. The migrants' issues were often difficult to identify, control and maintain given the limitations of both ship size and crew numbers. Multiple medical conditions, near drownings and second-degree burns were all difficult to treat and we'd often be overwhelmed in a short period of time.

Tensions within the migrants rescued were raised at times for a variety of reasons including hunger, dehydration, pain, trauma, missing family members, language barriers and conflict. Many different nationalities were rescued, all with many different reasons for leaving their countries. The furthest recorded on our mission was Nepal. Commonly, individuals sought refuge from Afghanistan, Iraq, Syria, Liberia, Sierra Leone, Ethiopia, Somalia, and Sudan.

The ship operated red and green zones for the personnel attached to the ship – green zone being the area inside where personnel took their rest. The main deck was the red zone, comprising accommodation, a field medical station, and sanitary areas. The ship's company operated on a four-hour rotation of staff for the two-day repatriation, as conditions were difficult for ship members as well: white HAZMAT suits[34] with N95 masks,[35] double gloves and goggles were worn. Temperatures exceeding 40°C made the role extremely difficult, sweat, chafing, and wrinkly fingers causing discomfort, especially during the active rescue phases of the operation.

During the transit back to Sicily, strict security and medical observations were maintained, liaising with Italian Red Cross and Interpol for criminal elements and further medical treatment pathways. Numerous factors had to be considered as embarkation commenced. Potential threats such as terrorist activity, diseases like Ebola and dysentery, public order concerns, and the presence of rival factions from war-torn countries all added complexity to the situation. With up to 600 people on the deck enduring uncomfortable conditions during the two-day repatriation period, tensions could escalate. Upon disembarkation in Sicily, we would transit to Malta to resupply, restock, clean, and prepare for the next deployment in three days' time.

This was the routine: two weeks of duty followed by three days of rest in the beautiful city of Valletta, Malta, then back to duty at sea for another two weeks. This cycle repeated over a three-month period. I cannot quantify the number of individuals I assisted during that summer, but what I do know is that nearly 1200 men, women, and children lost their lives at sea that year. Sadly, the situation has not improved since then.

Niall Carty
Lecturer in Paramedic Science
Military Naval Rescue; Education

Some people see

Some people see what it's like to be
a paramedic in society.
A happy smile and a caring face,
they see you there, to replace
the upset, the anger,
the frustration and panic;
We turn up on scene when it's absolutely frantic.
They see you make a difference with your knowledge and skills,
to the patients' condition
when they're really ill.

Some people don't see the reality,
as a paramedic in society.
They don't see the upset, they don't see the fear.
They don't see the frustration, or the anger that is near.
They don't see the policies, nor the procedures,
they don't see the statistics that are there between us.
They don't see the rules, or the regulations,
the HCPC guidelines[36] or the accusations.

Some people don't see inside of me,
as a paramedic in society.
They don't see my upset, they don't see my tears,
they don't see my frustrations; they don't know my fears.
They don't see my stress, nor my anxiety,
they don't know my job or see the variety.
They don't see me when I get home from work;
it might have been a good shift, it might have had perks.
It might have been a bad one, I might feel hurt.
Every job we don't know what we'll see,
I need a coping mechanism to look after me.

I use self-havening and meditation,
gratitude, better words with positive thinking.
I try to only look at the present moment,
I don't look back, or very far forwards,
the past has gone with the future to arrive,
being present is here *it is good to be alive.*

A feeling is a thought with emotions attached,
I now take an image and remove the bad,
I remove the colour turn it black and white,
remove the sound and shrink it till it's downsized;
I then replace the image with a positive memory,
increase the size increasing positivity.

Perhaps you can now see inside of me,
as a paramedic in society.
I walk into work with a smile on my face,
knowing it's only my mind getting in my way.
The job itself isn't difficult to do,
But you NEED a coping mechanism, to look after YOU.

Kirsty Wood
Paramedic
Ambulance Services

Zero to one hundred

My crewmate was what is affectionately known in the service as a "shit magnet".[37] It had been a hectic shift thus far, marked by two contrasting but significant calls: one celebrating new life with a successful birth (both mother and baby doing well), and the other grappling with a cardiac arrest, where we terminated on scene with the patient surrounded by their loved ones. The next call seemed benign – a 13-year-old child with a headache. You get the mundane with the extreme.

This call was unusual though – the teenager had had a sudden onset of a headache the day before, which had developed with dizziness and vomiting over the day. Our examination showed nothing of significance, and it had the hallmark features of a migraine, rather than meningitis, but something was amiss. We were discussing options for further investigation; the teenager began to grow increasingly drowsy – a concerning development. Initially responsive to voice, then to pain, his condition took a worrisome turn.

As my crewmate retrieved the stretcher from the ambulance, the teenager's condition rapidly deteriorated. In the blink of an eye, he went from zero to one hundred, experiencing a full tonic-clonic seizure.[38] Though the seizure subsided on its own, it left him in a decerebrate posture – a concerning position where the arms and legs extend straight out, toes point downward, and the head and neck arch backwards. This posture is typically associated with severe brain damage.

We gave the only thing we could do: diesel. An emergency drive through the streets of the city (hence the diesel) to the nearest paediatric emergency department, where we were received by a team of consultants and nurses.

I've no idea what happened after that. We cleared and were sent to the next job: a female under a train. There's nothing mundane about our profession.

Anonymous

Finding the essence of being a paramedic

Sheltering on the bottom bunk, I was absolutely terrified. Tropical cyclone Harold was producing a wind speed of 350 km/h along with half a metre of rain in six hours. Parts of the roof had been lost, water was coming in in many places and the floor was covered in 100 mm of water. The walls were literally shaking, and the roof had hit a resonant frequency so loud that it drowned out the scream of the wind outside.

Outside, whole sheets of corrugated iron were flying past the windows, travelling so fast that when they hit a tree they stuck in and started to make a screaming noise of their own. Indeed, some trees had given up and were literally flying towards the sea having come out of the ground with their roots still intact.

I had travelled to a remote island in the South Pacific to teach three paramedic students. I arrived, as a volunteer, on the day that the World Health Organization declared coronavirus disease (COVID-19) a pandemic. I had volunteered initially to teach for two months, but had become marooned on the island. We had no COVID-19, but when the time to return came round there were no flights and no ships. The Australian paramedics, all volunteers, had had to return to Australia on the last flights. Not being an Australian, I had no option but to stay and gladly agreed to run the ambulance service on the island along with my students. One week later cyclone Harold had arrived and quite literally destroyed the island.

With a long career working for three different ambulance services in the UK, as well as volunteering in several hot, poor, and difficult places, I had experience of several major incidents. This was different; I had never been a victim as well as rescuer. Our two ambulances had survived, but to start with there were very few roads that we could actually drive on. There was no electricity, water, or any telecommunications. What is more, we were not allowed to have any help. The lack of COVID-19 in the islands meant we were in isolation.

The next three weeks were very hard, both physically and emotionally. On a personal level I had doubts as to whether I would ever get home. I had spent a lot of time away from home in the past but had always known my date of return. As the only paramedic I was continuously on call 24 hours a day. In fact, it would be seven months before I was able to leave the island and I had been on call for all that time. My students stepped up to the mark and made sure that they didn't disturb me unnecessarily – but my clinical responsibility hung heavy on my shoulders.

Being a paramedic on an island in the South Pacific is quite challenging. The number of calls is not particularly high, but those that you do get can take a long time to complete. The island was the size of a large English county, with the one road that went 20 miles to the west coast taking three hours to drive in an emergency. There were four large rivers to ford along with some steep hills that were either muddy or rocky. Even when electricity was restored there was very little light after dark. Getting out of the vehicle at night, you could commonly expect large bats to brush your hair, huge coconut crabs to challenge you, along with the dangers of packs of wild dogs and the occasional wild pig.

The case mix is very different. In the tropics, wounds are much more problematic, and the prevalence of type II diabetes also means that dressing skills have got to be good for chronic wound management. The infectious conditions that are seen are certainly different. Leptospirosis, dengue fever, tuberculoma and Guillain–Barré are all common. Child deaths are upsetting wherever they happen but when you have scarce resources and no back-up, it is hard not to be overwhelmed.

I had plenty of time to think. No television, no social media. I had quite quickly read all the books available to me. I felt very privileged. In that time, I understood the essence of being a paramedic. Whilst there are great advantages in paramedics accessing pathways and signposting patients, I had been in a position where I had to deal with what was in front of me. The challenges were what kept me going. There were lots of things which I could have done better, but I can rest easy in the knowledge that I didn't fail.

I left the UK on 1 February and didn't return until October two years later. The return journey was long, and certainly not simple, but nothing like as hard as readapting to being a paramedic back in the NHS.

Nich Woolf
Paramedic
Ambulance Services

Butterflies

When my radio crackles to life, I feel the initial flutter of butterflies until I've connected with control. Once I have the details, I'm swiftly on my way to the given address. With my role as a postman and my life-long residency in the community, I often know the individuals I'm attending. For me, there's nothing quite like the relief of seeing the ambulance and paramedics arrive. By that time, I've already taken some initial vital signs and gained valuable insights into the situation, which I can then pass on to them.

Contributing to my community in this capacity fills me with immense pride, and I'm honoured to collaborate with such exceptional professionals. Their dedication and resilience in the face of daily challenges are truly admirable. It's remarkable to witness them seamlessly transition from their demanding work to their personal lives.

Having served as a community first responder for eleven years, I can confidently say that this experience has shaped me profoundly, and much of that credit goes to the unwavering support of the incredibly skilled individuals who work in the ambulance service. Try as you might, you won't convince me otherwise!

Craig Lusk
Volunteer Community First Responder and Postman
Ambulance Services

A tipsy mess

The job drops down on the mobile data terminal:[22] 80-year-old female, welfare check after alarm activation.

This is a standard job that we get often and normally the patient has hit the alarm button by accident and is confused as to why we are there. Arriving on scene, it takes us a moment to get into the upmarket building, which we note is supported retirement accommodation, and to the flat door. The door to the flat is slightly ajar, but we knock anyway. No answer. It's dark inside. I hear some noise coming from behind the door; I push it open gently, announcing our arrival.

"Oh no, is that blood?" my crewmate asks. I follow her eyes to the dark-coloured stains on the walls and floor. I take a sniff. "Oh, nope that's poo."

It transpired our patient had attended a party at a neighbouring flat and had consumed an inordinate amount of red wine. On returning to the flat, she'd had several episodes of explosive diarrhoea which she had initially taken to be flatulence from the rich meal and wine. Still tipsy, and now covered unexpectedly in her own poop, she'd slipped and pulled onto the alarm in the bathroom in an effort to stay upright as she attempted to clean herself up.

She alternated between embarrassment and giggles as we helped her to shower and made an effort to clean the poo off the walls and floor in the hallway.

Sometimes the job can be messy, sometimes smelly, and sometimes not what I thought I would be doing when I qualified as a paramedic. But when the patient is as lovely as this giggly tipsy 80-year-old lady, who was still living her life and enjoying a party, it makes it worthwhile.

Emma Jane Briggs
Paramedic
Ambulance Services

Privilege

In the space of twelve hours:

I met a child, five years after I helped deliver and resuscitate them at birth.

And shook the hand of a man that was clinically dead 30 minutes before.

This job has its moments and today was one of them.

Being a paramedic is a privilege.

Anonymous

All is fine

I have offered my condolences to a thousand grieving loved ones,
I have seen the wicked things people do with knives and with shotguns.
I have volunteered to be the lasting memory for parents learning their child has departed,
my voice, my face, my words leave them forever broken-hearted.
Without back-up I have delivered twin babies, both dead,
as I kneel in the blood loss from their mother staining me red.
Dismembered and broken bodies are now normal to smell and see,
my eyes have viewed so many, how good can this be?
I have held the hand of a lonely man as he takes his last breath,
I have looked into his frightened eyes before that final moment of rest.
I have ghosts on every street from the catalogue of triple nine calls,
the three-year-old hanging, the 21-year-old asthma – I remember them all.
My trusty clipboard has supported me writing thousands of tragic reports,
as I reflect on my performance and collect my thoughts.
Sixty years of happy marriage end at the time that I declare,
I speak to the now wifeless husband and feel his despair.
Some scream, some cry, and some stare with nothing to say,
their life, their love, their heart and soul, has been taken away.
Blue lights and sirens, racing to the next patient just in time,
a success, a happy story. Peace is restored and all is fine.

Scott Hardy
Critical Care Team Leader (Paramedic)
Ambulance Services

NIGHT SHIFT

The night shift

Darkness, a vulnerable place. I wander to patrol my mind.

The streets, soulless, the buzz of the day lost to the "nee-naw" of night.

They approached. I saw their story reflected in their eyes by the neon light.

I reached for your gloved hand. Human to human we understood.

Karen Scott
Lecturer and Simulation Lead for Paramedic Program
Education

Click

Click... The familiar aroma filling all my senses all at once. Overwhelming. Pain. Trauma. Grief.

All at once a flash, click, click, click, playing out in slow motion.

In seconds, transported back to that road. Heat, oil, fumes, sweat. A mix of human bodies scrambling in the night.

A cold autumnal evening. A finish time of 7 pm, resting on station at five to six. A welcome and unusual reprise towards the end of a busy day covering many miles. Tired, hungry, and weary with aching bones. The kettle had started to boil, a rare treat of a hot cup of tea out of an actual kettle. What a gift. We chatted about the television programme playing in the background on the old square grey TV in the corner that went fuzzy every now and again. The end was in sight.

I had started to close my heavy tired hot eyes, when that all-too-familiar bleep rang out. The radio. Our friend and foe.

Category 1[5] – RTC[39] – car versus van. A few miles from the station.

The usual surge of adrenaline started to fill my body as we scrambled into the cab. Dusk was drizzling and chilly, causing a yearning for the hot cup of tea left undrunk on the side in the crew room. Chart music blasted out of the radio, in and out of reception as we turned the corner into the narrow single-carriageway road. I didn't hear it at all as we approached the scene up ahead, music replaced by shouting and yelling, with lots of waving. The public. They were yelling and screaming at us to help. A fire engine approached from the opposite direction.

Between us, two vehicles were crumpled into each other.

That is when I saw him, illuminated in the half-light of dusk and the mix of blue lights between fire engine and ambulance.

His face.

His shirt.

The crisp white shirt. His skin. Perfect and youthful. Handsome. Someone's friend. Someone's fiancé. Someone's son.

I instructed my crewmate to see to the driver of the other vehicle. I started to breathe more heavily as I ran towards the other, one of those small car-cum-van type vehicles.

His face was white.

I tried to drag him out myself. He was wedged under the steering wheel. His neck was cold, I couldn't feel a pulse. I quickly instructed the firefighters to help me drag him out. Instructions were passed quickly between them as they organised equipment swiftly and efficiently.

My voice caught in my throat as I talked to him, the vehicle a barrier between us. His face. His face that would haunt my dreams, and still brings tears to my eye even now as I write this five years on.

His face was perfect. No scratch. Just perfect and untouched. His eyes though. His eyes will forever be etched into my soul. They were fixed. Staring. In horror. In fear. In utter terrified shock.

That's when I noticed it. The scent. A familiar popular aftershave. Favoured by the young males who doused themselves regularly on shift, or similarly on a night out. The comforting wafts of youth. All at once, images of what he would be like as a person, and not just a body, flashed before my eyes. A picture developed right in front of me.

A white shirt soaked in aftershave, dating, or a recent engagement perhaps. A loved son. A mother full of worry. A dad proud of his achievements. A hard-working lad earning his own money and learning his craft. A trade. A reliable bloke. A mate. A laugh. A few pints. Click, click, click. Images one after the other came in and out of focus.

His jeans under the steering wheel looked new. Crisp and ironed. Boots shiny. Trying to impress, I thought. As we pulled him out finally, the white expensive shirt cut off into pieces, the smell hit me once again. Off out. Dinner? Perhaps home after dinner and an afternoon out.

I tried. I tried so hard.

Cue utter frustration and helplessness. His airway. No. Please no. Please work. Please. A gush of continuous brown liquid surged, causing the iGel[40] to bob up like a little buoy on the sea.

The smell. The familiar smell of digesting food. He'd just eaten. A nice meal? A nice memory made. Love shared. Conversation and laughter with every mouthful. Suction unit. Please help him. Please. Clonk. That all too familiar noise of the tubing. Clonk. Blocked. Try something else. Try this. Try that. No pulse. Try again. Sweat. Blood. Vomit. Rain. Try again. And again. And again. Rhythm check after rhythm check. PLEASE.

STOP. Ceased resuscitation at...

Rain. Pain. Tears. Sweat. Soaked through to the bones.

The shirt. His jeans still with his wallet in the pocket. The socks he put on that morning. The shaving cut he caused with the razor. The eyes. Fixed.

He will be getting cold. Let's wrap him up all nice.

I tried. I really did.

Kaitee Robinson
Senior Lecturer and Paramedic
Education and Ambulance Services

Unconditional

Where did it go
that youthful blow
which contained such a glow

When did you look so old
So frail with such detail

The frayed rug on the floor
walked over by all
And now we lie here
ignored
where life once poured

So you look out of the window
and dream of a place you would rather be
For I will never love more than thee

I shall look after you now
My love
until you fly away
For I shall meet you that day

So I shall clasp your hand and think of
our vows and tut as to where all the guests are now

And I will administer the pills for the pain so you don't
wane and fade like the rain

For the clouds won't leave

and we will never part

For you are forever lodged in my heart.

Natalie Sallis
Apprentice Paramedic
Emergency Care

Eighteen minutes

As a student paramedic, I always wanted to go to the interesting, weird, wonderful, and sometimes scary jobs for the adrenaline and experience. I challenge any student that would deny this. It wasn't until years later that I realised the impact these adrenaline-fuelled incidents could have on a clinician. Looking back now, one job stuck with me as a student that opened my eyes to the unexpected and harrowing nature that can sometimes come with our role in the ambulance services.

It was a bitter winter evening. My mentor, their crewmate and I were getting a coffee from the fabulous BP garages that offer discount to emergency services, having a well-deserved five-minute break before the next job came in. My mentor and I had a reputation for not being called to the most challenging cases; in other words, we were the antithesis of "shit magnets".[37] A category 1[5] comes through as birth imminent on the mobile data terminal,[22] followed by an update stating it was a miscarriage. We knew this would be a highly emotive scene, which would need our ability to remain calm and provide reassurance and care for the mother – more than medical skills. On arrival at the address, we were met at the front gates by a man who confirmed he was husband and father. In a frantic manner, he stated it was a miscarriage and the dead baby was born in the toilet. Perhaps it was in response to his evident panic, but unspoken we decided to bring a considerable amount of equipment into the property. In hindsight, I recognise this was the instinctual feeling clinicians experience when something doesn't quite add up, a sentiment reflected in the expressions of both my mentor and crewmates.

Navigating to the bathroom, we found the mother sat still on the toilet, a look of shock on her face. Without delay, but with reassurance and calm, we supported her to stand and move away from the toilet. In doing so we found a baby, full term, lying still underwater in the bowl of the toilet. Motionless. The placenta was stuck to the ceramic just above the water line. As my mentor and crewmate had a quick discussion to prepare to extricate the baby safely from the toilet, I recognised the harrowing sound of gargling. Drowning. It was evident at this point that the baby was not only born in the toilet but was currently drowning. The urgency was also heightened on realising that the mother had been sat on the toilet for 8 minutes and it took us as a crew 10 minutes to get to the address on lights and sirens. The baby had been underwater 18 minutes.

It took two of us to safely extricate the baby and the placenta from the toilet. Something I would have nightmares about for some time to come. The baby was grey and remained lifeless with the occasional gasp of air. Agonal breathing. My mentor called for help, requesting Helicopter Emergency Medical Services[41] (HEMS), critical care paramedics[42] (CCPs) and in all honesty, any help we could get. The overwhelming demand on the service became apparent – HEMS was occupied with another task, there were no CCPs available, and no crews were in close proximity. It was just the three of us.

We started down the neonatal life support algorithm, starting with rescue breaths. Mirrored in each other's eyes were our mutual expressions of hope and despair. Hope that we may get the baby to breathe again, but despair on knowing the likelihood of this was slim. All of a sudden, a cry. A beautiful cry of relief. The best cry I have ever heard in my life to this date. Grey turned to pink, each still, lifeless limb began moving and filled with life, blood and oxygen. I think this was the first time I breathed.

With no other resources available, we conveyed mother and baby together (normally they would travel separately to benefit from dedicated care by a paramedic). At the hospital, we were greeted by a mixture of about 15 doctors and nurses – their disbelief clear at the arrival of a pink baby following our pre-alert and description of what happened.

My mentor congratulated me for hearing the gargling of the baby underwater. As a student, you strive for feedback, for compliments when you've done the right thing. However, at that time, I just wanted silence and time, needing to process what had happened and what we as a team had accomplished. I stepped out. I didn't feel accomplished, happy, or proud of myself. I felt distraught for the child, mother, father, and their whole family, despite the positive and very surprising outcome. The dump of adrenaline hit me hard.

As rain poured outside the hospital, I found myself overwhelmed by a wave of emotions that felt too heavy to bear alone. In that moment, all I wanted was to hear the comforting voices of my family. They had always assured me that they would be there for me whenever I needed them. So, I called my mum and dad, and as soon as I heard their familiar voices, tears welled up in my eyes. Knowing that my family, who knew me better than anyone else, could offer the solace I sought, I gathered the strength to return to the hospital and finish the rest of my shift.

Reflecting on my experiences, I've learned to anticipate the unexpected in the incidents we respond to and to avoid becoming too complacent in our work. One moment that will forever stay with me is returning to the hospital after receiving some heartfelt advice from my parents, and visiting the new mother and her newborn baby. As I looked into the mother's eyes, she expressed her gratitude, saying "If it wasn't for you recognising my baby was breathing, if it wasn't for you, I wouldn't have a daughter".

Abigail Tucker
Newly Qualified Paramedic
Ambulance Services

What they don't teach you

It was a welfare check – a call for someone who had not been seen for some time. We were met at the front door by the police, who kicked it in so hard they broke the lock. There was no response as we called out into the tidy, warm flat. The front door slammed shut behind us.

It looked like he'd just rolled out of bed, resting in the narrow space between the side of the bed and the radiator on the wall of his bedroom. I hoped his death had been more peaceful than his decomposition. The heat of the radiator had caused his head to melt into his neck, his cervical vertebrae glistening under his residue skin in a partial decapitation. He'd been in that position for so long, even the flies had moved on to a fresher meal.

It had been a terrible accident, and I hope he had been dead long before the radiator came on. Nothing in my paramedic degree had prepared me for such a sight, but you find a way to work through it, complete your paperwork, and move on to the next call.

Will Broughton
Professor of Paramedicine
Education

A story of three parts: the elephant on the road

Part A: The encounter

CALL
Handover wrapped up, tidy back of the truck. Peep through the pigeonhole and wait.
Debate greening up, mobile data terminal[22] instantly erupts: CARDIAC/RESPIRATORY ARREST, 2 YEARS.
Crew in denial and casual, sirens swarm the streets. Sit stunned in silence each bend we meet.
ETA: 3 MINUTES.

ARRIVE
Reverse-park into a bay, mentor bolts away, grab any kit and follow through.
Cross the lawn towards the doorway, little girls bawling with tears.
Mum's worst fears, instructions over loudspeaker. We appear, she begs us to take over.

AT SCENE
Her face lay pale, lips stained and stale, eyes partially open. Hand on her heart we begin.
Switch on the LifePak,[43] fingers fumble shears, pads attached.
Cycle through rhythms, airway suctioned, calm with compressions.
Insert tube, auscultate[13] her lungs, quick plan, scoop and go.

LEAVE SCENE
Quick carry through the door, in the back we go.
Lay her down, stroke her crown. VENTILATE.
Grab the EZ-IO,[44] hold her leg, and drill.

RESUS
Roll up and reverse like we always rehearse.
Where is the team?
Met by a young teen on her own, rush into resus.
Slide across, handover delayed, we stay and play.
Bedlam ensues in the beehive as people stream in.
Mayhem. Chaos. Frantic. Disorder.
An hour flies by, I look Mum in the eyes and ask her child's name.
Write it on the wall, now we all know.

HANDOVER COMPLETE
Open the door, look to the floor. See the stretcher, take a seat.
The roars of resus drown, the silence returns. And breathe.
What just happened?

Part B: The vision

It was my eleventh shift in my first year as a student paramedic, second call of my night shift, and I attended my first cardiac arrest. My experience has come to define me in many ways. With time and experience, I CHOSE to let it empower and inspire me. To learn more about myself, the people around me, those we care for, and explore how we improve the way we perform as practitioners.

This journey has driven me to ask questions people will think of yet are afraid to ask, discuss topics we rarely talk about yet know all too well. I call it "the elephant on the road".

In a rapidly changing world, I continue to see the patterns, trends, and rich intricate detail. With new challenges and crises arise opportunities, but too often I have felt many are unwilling to heed and substantively act. Feelings, ideas, experiences frequently dismissed.

But I CHOOSE not to dismiss them. I CHOOSE to listen and learn. I CHOOSE to find a way to contribute to our practice, to enhance our well-being and performance, however long it takes.

Part C: The journey

I start with myself, then grow from here.

Being a paramedic is one of myriad ways I can draw upon my various streams of experience to contribute to the world around me, particularly via my own platform, drBACKPACK. I am lucky to have forged a path featuring countless diverse contexts and settings, and to have opportunities to do things in my own way – forms that reflect my values and identity. I feel privileged and grateful to be there for people in their time of need, and what's exciting is I'm only just getting started.

My journey continues.

Wasim Ahmed
Paramedic, Academic, Educator, Artist, Adventurer
and Volunteer
DrBACKPACK

COVID – the fight as a paramedic

It was a cold night when I got the call
my first COVID patient, fallen in a long cold hall.
Babbling and mumbling in PPE
to focus with grace was absent in me.

In a haze of fear, dexterity had gone
bubbling like a lobster in my own hot pan.
An uncomfortable heat steamed in me,
face to face with the virus – it was COVID, you see.

Listening to a chest, our breaths as one.
This virus was lurid; in silence, it stung.
In and out and irregularly fast.
The family's first words, "Is it COVID?" they gasped.

The fear in those eyes was solemn and deep,
nebs[24] and IVs[26] were indeed a feat.
Above in the light, a murmuration like sleet,
droplets were falling in a room that was neat.

The conversion of fear in this room all alone,
the monitor beeps on a hand with no tone.
Words are essential, just like a hymn –
precise and purposeful – "She needs to go in".

Leads are cluttered as I doff alone
whilst I look to the stars and wonder of home.
On a rain-soaked night, the heavens look numb,
as I remember the faces of these days that are glum.

Death is more frequent
with tasks that are slow.
I squat with a pen
and an old sweaty glow.

Within our team, we're gathered as one
"How are you doing?" is a question from some.
Clinical outcomes are debriefed and discussed,
we're in it together – we don't need to combust.
Community and family have been our support,
yet we must walk as clinicians into clusters unsought.
It's our duty to help the fallen and meek
all alone in these siren-filled streets.

So who cares for the carers on anxious-filled lanes?
Or the tired and bewildered who'll perform once again.
The sting of COVID runs deep like a sin.
What we do to recover has reshaped us to win.

On this frost-bitten night.
I recall some Latin of life:
In omnia paratus –
be prepared in all things.

I shall remember them all.
Till the day that I fall.

Adrian McGrath
Clinical Support Paramedic
Ambulance Services

Call me superstitious

Working in the ambulance service is just so varied, and you never know what you will be sent to next. But some dates, and some circumstances, can be more predictably unpredictable than most.

It was Friday the 13th, and a full moon was expected. This nightshift started like any other: arrive, meet your crewmate and mentor, sign onto the vehicle, do a kit check, and then we're off. We had a lovely start to the evening, with several calls to local care homes, the residents of which were well and gave us the opportunity to start our shift with plenty of chatter, tea, and cake.

It was almost midnight; we'd just discharged our patient and were wrapping up our paperwork whilst enjoying a supper of tea and scones when the radio went off. High-speed RTC.[39] Category 2.[4] We weren't far from the location and were first on scene. It was a "big" job – four passengers, all my age, each with significant injuries. We were supported by police and fire crews, as well as a critical care paramedic. As a student paramedic, I worked alongside my mentor but as part of a much larger team – each contributing skills and experience to deliver successful patient outcomes.

On clearing the hospital, we all went back to base to have a debrief. I'll forever be grateful for these moments, as they're not just isolated incidents. There's always someone there to check in on you after these challenging assignments, and that small gesture can make all the difference. By now, it was the early hours of the morning, the moon so bright there was no need for streetlamps.

We'd finished our debrief alongside another cup of tea, and alerted control to our availability. We were immediately sent another job. Thirty-four-year-old male, stiletto in rectum. Talk about unpredictability, we laughed. It would be one of those shifts.

This shift demonstrated the three things I love most about the ambulance service: support, superstition, and humour. I think it would be hard to be a paramedic without this.

Anonymous

A community of hands working together

I work in Northern Ireland as a clinical support paramedic officer with the Northern Ireland Ambulance Service and have 25 years of experience as a paramedic infused into the heart of my soul. I'm sharing with you a story where I witnessed colleagues from both emergency and non-emergency tiers, along with local community first responders, collaborating to assist a patient in cardiac arrest. This experience left me inspired, highlighting the remarkable potential we possess when working together during high-acuity calls in unfamiliar settings.

It was after 9 o'clock on a damp, chilly evening, with raindrops bouncing off the asphalt under the ambulance's headlights. We'd been dispatched to a 69-year-old male who had called with chest pain. The blue lights cast an eerie glow, illuminating the hedges lining both sides of the road, when our data terminal updated that he was now in cardiac arrest. That fragile tide of life had stopped beating in this patient. The rain shimmered in the lights, casting a surreal spectrum of colours as we drove through the downpour. Such weather added an extra layer of difficulty to driving under emergency conditions, the vehicle's wipers and the driver's eyes worked seamlessly together to focus on the demands of getting there safely and on time. A discernible shift in focus occurred, evident as condensation formed on the windows due to heightened respiratory rates and the release of cortisol into the capillaries. Our conversation shifted, replaced by a sense of hypervigilance characterised by a stern focus on driving and a shared mental model of our approach to the patient upon arrival.

As we entered the street, our blue lights cast reflections off the windows of the houses lining both sides, revealing shadows of neighbours waving us down and signalling for us to follow them further along the road. If you know, you know. It was as given. Light spilled out of an open front door, cars parked haphazardly, an upstairs bedroom.

Cardiopulmonary resuscitation was actively in progress by two patient care support staff and a community first responder; the first two links in the chain of survival (CPR and defibrillation) were activated. There was still hope. In one breath, the community volunteers gave a seamless handover – they'd been with the patient following the first emergency call for chest pain and the patient collapsed in their presence. We were only five minutes behind them. They had been prompt in starting chest compressions and applying the defibrillator pads, subsequently giving two shocks[53] prior to our arrival. This was good news, this was positive, I nodded as they talked. Early CPR had been initiated, and our clinical team integrated with the volunteers, operating through seamless efficiency, with a calm and focused demeanour. It was akin to a symphony of precision; a sense of harmony pervaded the room. While it may sound sentimental, the clinical synergy among the team was palpable. Experienced hands worked in perfect synchronisation, resulting in the patient's positive response after the fifth shock.

Encouragingly, new indicators emerged, prompting a shift towards situational awareness and the delegation of new tasks. The patient began showing signs of return of spontaneous circulation[3] indicating a low-flow state.[45] However, intensive clinical care was now imperative. Drawing on the paramedics' clinical experience, tasks were assigned and executed calmly and supportively. Intermittent positive pressure ventilation[46] was administered to support the patient's breathing and reassess airway patency.[47] Intravenous access[26] remained patent, and end-tidal CO_2[48] levels showed promising signs. A sense of quiet relief permeated the small back bedroom, underscoring the significance of the moment. Medication was administered to increase blood pressure and fluids to bolster intravascular volume[49] and support kidney function. Allowing the patient time to stabilise was crucial for self-sustained perfusion.[50] Ten minutes later, we undertook a tracing of his heart, confirming that he had had a heart attack, and we contacted the local hospital's cardiology team. During this interim period, the team collectively absorbed the gravity of their actions, briefly contemplating the extrication process after successfully resuscitating the patient. He was responding to our treatment, and we now needed to ensure he could be seen by the specialist team that could fix the problem that had caused his cardiac arrest.

Allow me to segue into discussing the dynamics of teamwork that unfolded that night.

Five individuals had directly contributed to this patient's survival: two clinicians and three community volunteers. Like the interconnected roots of a tree, there was a seamless cohesion among us, maintaining balance, focus, and performance as we worked together towards our objective. With one leader calmly directing the process, we worked in unison, each contributing to the task at hand. It was a privilege to witness such synchronised teamwork, filling me with pride for our profession. Even after 25 years, witnessing colleagues operate with such efficiency still resonates deeply with me. It's a genuine honour to fulfil this role, stepping into strangers' homes, collaborating seamlessly with unfamiliar faces, and orchestrating life-saving treatment amidst the emotional turmoil of the patient's loved ones leaning on us for support.

It was a community of hands working together. This model of working is so crucial to promote calmness and structure. In the bustling world of prehospital care, one must have a situational awareness – taking note of the furniture arrangement, winding stairs and any potential hazards like loose carpets or pets underfoot. All whilst treating the patient and managing the expectations of the family. There is so much to process, manage and review. Crafted over years of experience, this artistry is the hallmark of an effective team, whether composed of community first responders or seasoned ambulance professionals. While clinical expertise forms the backbone of their practice, it's the nuanced interplay of communication, social finesse, and empathetic awareness that truly elevates their performance. These skills are not taught on university courses or in textbooks, but honed through countless encounters and interactions. They are the invisible threads that weave through every aspect of the scene, shaping its dynamic and contributing to the broader clinical narrative. Without them, the picture would be incomplete, lacking the human touch that defines compassionate care.

Human factors are paramount in such situations, demanding a deliberate effort to regulate one's breathing and maintain vigilance over the surroundings. It's a delicate balance, remaining attuned to drug dosages, clinical procedures, and the performance of colleagues while navigating hazards like vomit on the floor, which can complicate even the most routine tasks. When all these elements align, when every member of the team is fully engaged and aware, magic happens. No egos or distractions, just a pure genuine focus on teamwork that allows everyone to perform at their absolute best when it matters most.

Let us return to our patient that night.

Extricating the patient presented its own set of challenges. Given the delicate nature of the patient's vascular compromise and blood pressure, we opted to keep him flat. Once again, all our hands acted with a unified determination. Under the calm guidance, each member was assigned a specific task. Their response of "tell us what you need, and we will do it" epitomised the teamwork required in such situations. The scene unfolded like a perfectly orchestrated wave, with a seamless flow of constructive action, confirmation of instruction, and reassurance to the patient – who remained unresponsive but alive.

Remaining grounded and quickly acknowledging one's team is essential in this role. Through simple introductions and maintaining a calm demeanour, we build vital working relationships and recognise each person's unique skill set as a crucial link in the chain. This cohesive teamwork is instrumental in achieving the ultimate goal: restoring the patient to a fully functional state, just as they were before the medical emergency occurred.

The exemplary work witnessed that night has served as my benchmark for achieving excellence on high-acuity calls. It involves uplifting team members, providing constructive feedback and in some cases fostering authentic learning opportunities. These moments are pivotal for shaping the standards and practices of future paramedics. By prioritising evidence-based practice and maintaining situational awareness of human factors, we consistently make a positive impact on our patients' lives.

In this case, our patient went on to have a successful outcome and returned home to his family some months later. Every now and then, I spot him strolling through town, offering a subtle nod of his head towards the ambulance, a gesture filled with appreciation and respect for our work.

Adrian McGrath
Clinical Support Paramedic
Ambulance Services

Connections

I could write a thousand stories of my 20 years in the ambulance service, but there are two that I would call career-defining – connected in a way I couldn't have foreseen.

Whilst this shift was more than 15 years ago, it feels like it was only last week. We were working a weekend night shift. It was one of those autumn nights, the air was fresh, moist, and there was a light fog as we drove through the mostly quiet rural streets. The shift had been busy, and we hadn't long finished our very overdue meal break when we were dispatched to a collision: car vs tree.

Approaching the scene, we were met by a blanket of blue lights from our police and fire colleagues. Debris littered the road up to the mangled, smoking wreck up ahead. There was very little urgency on scene, which indicates one of two things: either a poor prognosis for the patients involved, or the crumple zones of the vehicles have done their job and the passengers are miraculously fine. We could see from the faces of the police officers who greeted us as we parked that it was the former in this case. The car of four had been travelling at speed before hitting a kerb and coming to rest wrapped round the trunk of a tree. The car had hit the tree with such force that the engine was found 20 ft further down the road in a neighbouring tree, and the driver and front passenger were facing each other feet to feet on the other side of the tree to the rear of the car. Death would have been instant for the front two male passengers. In the rear of the car had sat two women. One, no more than 20 years old, was clearly deceased, her neck at such an angle that it caused her head to rest on the neighbouring seat's headrest. The other rear passenger was out of the car and, miraculously, alive. She'd not been ejected; she had climbed out of the smashed rear window and had been attempting to drag herself away from the smoking wreckage when the first fire engine arrived. She had obvious, open, bloody fractures to both legs. We took over from the firefighters who had provided initial casualty management, splinted her legs, and stabilised her for transport. A police car escorted us to the nearest emergency department.

Handover and paperwork completed, we were made unavailable for any other emergencies in the area and sent back to our station to debrief and grab a cuppa.

We hadn't been at station long when control called us – there was an outstanding call for a male who had collapsed, could we attend? Could we have done with a little longer to debrief and decompress after the horrific accident we'd just attended? Yes. But an emergency is an emergency, and our role is to preserve life... so we accepted. At the end of the day, we are an emergency service so these sights should be expected... right?

Back in the cab of the ambulance, I looked at the incident address as my crewmate flickered the ignition back into life. Odd. The location was just round the corner from the fatal collision. We knew the road would still be closed for the police collision investigators to do their work, so we'd have to enter from the other side of the village. I asked control for further details of the call, to better prepare us to attend. Remembering the information given still sends as many chills through my veins today as it did on that night: "Male collapse. Police on scene. Has just received bad news". They didn't have any other details, but we felt it was too coincidental given the fatal crash earlier in the night.

We didn't need to check the address when we turned into the cul-de-sac of the incident address; it was the only house with the lights on in the now early hours of the morning, and a police car parked on the drive. We were met on the drive by one of the police officers who had attended our earlier call – the collapsed male was the father of the deceased driver. He had been told his son was involved in the crash and had immediately collapsed with chest pain. He was conscious and alert, but the police were rightly worried about him.

"Whatever you do, do not tell him you were on scene earlier," warned the police officer.

The atmosphere in the house was one that I never want to experience again. In the neat, orderly living room, a man was sitting in a chair, head held in his hands, sobbing. I knelt down in front of him, holding his hands in mine. For a brief moment, I had no idea what to say to him. Routine took over, and I introduced myself and my crewmate. From there, it was quickly established that the collapse was more emotional than physical. The reality was that there was nothing I could have said that would have made him worry about his own health needs anyway.

As we were navigating our clinical assessment, he asked us the question I had been willing him not to.

"... Did you go to my son?"

I wanted to say yes. I wanted to tell him that death for his son would have been instantaneous. That, at that time in my career, it was the worse car accident I had ever seen... I was spared from answering as, overcome by his grief, his sobs intensified. The pain in his eyes was palpable. Nothing quite prepares you for this sort of situation. No training manual, no supervision, no university course. He started talking about his son. So, we did the only thing we could do, we listened to him.

The next hour was probably the hardest of my professional career so far. This poor father proceeded to tell us all about who his son was. Not the one we had seen but the living one he had fathered for over 20 years. We were taken up to his bedroom to see his trophies, smell his aftershave. On the way back down the stairs, he explained the photos lined up on the hallway in detail. It was heart-breaking.

The connection between our attendance at the collision and being with his father, listening to the stories he shared with us of his son, took me to my emotional limit. I can't tell you how long we were on scene. When we eventually left, the man in the safe hands of the police's family liaison officer, in the safety of the cab of our ambulance my crewmate and I burst into tears.

On days like this, the only person who can really understand is the person you have shared the experience with. We consoled each other until the end of our shift, and many more shifts after that.

Do jobs like this make me regret my career path? Absolutely not.

Carrie Ingram
Frequent Caller Team Clinical Lead Paramedic
Ambulance Services

Time heals

Aged 18 and in my first year as a student paramedic. It was my first time away from my family, first time living alone, first time wearing a professional uniform... my first ambulance placement.

It was the middle of the night, rain pelting the roof of the ambulance. We were dispatched to a 'red one' – the terminology for cardiac arrest when I joined the service. I sat in the back of the ambulance on the way to the call, running through the various procedures in my head: 30:2 compressions, defibrillator on ASAP, grab the suction unit and a spare oxygen cylinder. I was prepared for this. University had drilled into us the "pit stop" approach and I felt prepared to face my first alongside my mentor and their crewmate. But when I walked into the dark address to find a young man hanging from a door frame by his dressing gown cord, every ounce of preparation left my body.

There are protocols to follow when you find someone obviously deceased and beyond help. We check for signs of life: do their pupils respond to light? We take a 30-second rhythm strip of their heart, checking if it's anything but still. And when it is, we tell their loved ones that the person has died.

I couldn't move. I was frozen in the hallway. At 18 years old, this was my first time seeing a dead body and I couldn't stop looking at the man's eyes. I knew this person was dead, his body was lifeless and pale but something behind the eyes just "wasn't there". That was the most unsettling thing. His soul had gone, and I felt like I could feel his sadness around the room. That sadness started to build up inside me.

All I wanted to do was leave. I was willing my mentor to say, "It's OK, you can wait outside," or "I'll do it, don't worry". Instead, he said simply, "You need to be here". At first, I wanted to burst into tears. I'd only seen dead bodies in horror films and my imagination was running away with itself. I felt my mentor's gentle encouragement as we moved through our checks to recognise life was extinct. I gently touched the man's jaw and lifted his arm... both were stiff, and he felt cold. But I did it, and nothing happened. Once that initial contact had been established, I was able to continue with the rest of the checks, albeit shakily.

I broke down crying on my way home whilst on the phone to my mum. Even now, a decade on, I can still remember the call vividly. I could walk around the house in my mind, I can picture the made bed, the photos of his family on the walls. I can still see his face. But it doesn't wake me at night any more and I don't start hyperventilating if I pass the address. I learned that time heals.

Time has desensitised me, and the faces of the deceased bother me less. I acknowledge that "something" has left them, and I always talk to them – I tell them what I'm doing whilst I do my checks, even though I know they can't hear me, but just in case that "something" is lingering around. But now I'm able to leave them behind, and they don't come home with me.

Jen Jackson
Paramedic
Ambulance Services

Heart sink

Navigating the world of the ambulance service can be daunting. The uncertainty about what lies ahead, the desire to make the correct decisions, and the fear of making mistakes can evoke a range of emotions. I experienced a whirlwind of feelings when dispatched to a paediatric cardiac arrest. Initially, I doubted it would truly be a cardiac arrest – how often do we respond to such calls for children only to find otherwise? Yet, my scepticism faded when the radio crackled to life, informing us that CPR had already commenced.

I was four months into my ambulance career and still what some would call "wet behind the ears". I was paired with a paramedic colleague who had a reputation for being difficult to work with. He was known on station for belittling new staff, rarely communicated with me, and scrutinised everything I did. Given the diverse range of people in the service, it's common to encounter colleagues we don't necessarily click with. This shift proved particularly challenging, as we struggled to establish rapport as a team. I found myself counting down the hours until the end of the shift, hoping to avoid working with that paramedic again.

We were due to finish at 01:30 and at midnight we got the call. It was out of our area so there was some distance to travel. As soon as I looked at the screen, my heart started racing. A cardiac arrest is the ultimate medical emergency, but a paediatric cardiac arrest, that was the ultimate, ultimate medical emergency. I was driving and my foot was already heavy on the accelerator as I was making my way up the motorway. The radio went and the dispatcher told us CPR had started. My foot became heavier on the accelerator, much to my disbelief that it was possible to get the ambulance up to the speed I was driving at. I had never driven as fast to a job as that night and haven't since.

I have also never run into a house before, but this one was different. I pulled up on the road outside the address, where I could see a lady waving at us, crying. Just behind us, the solo response vehicle was also pulling up. I jumped out from the driver's seat and grabbed what I could from the back of the ambulance. Taking the outside stairs two, three at a time, I followed my crewmate who was directed to an upstairs flat by the lady we'd seen on the road. It was her baby we were called to.

I burst through the front door following hot on the heels of my crewmate. Lying between the door frame of a bedroom and hallway, a father was kneeling over his three-month-old, carrying out chest compressions with two fingers on what looked like a training mannequin. My worst fear was realised. Her father looked up at us, tears flooding his face. My heart sank. Not only was this a paediatric cardiac arrest, I knew the father, I served time in the military with him, I knew his name. This provided an extra element for me – it became personal. We don't often attend people we know; we only find out names when we ask.

I took over compressions and my colleague applied the defibrillator pads... the screen showed us an unwavering flat line. Once an airway was established, I scooped the patient up and held her in my left arm. She was small enough that I could carry her in my arm and provide compressions with the other, all the while taking the stairs, this time three at a time going in the opposite direction. In the ambulance, we used an EZ-IO[44] drill to enable us to give medications into the patient's leg bone (as intravenous access[26] can be much more difficult in an emergency in a small child) and we started advanced life support. I was about to head back to the driver's seat when the patient's mum asked if she could go with us and she sat next to me in the front of the ambulance, her husband in the back with my two colleagues who were trying their best to revive her child.

As I drove to the hospital, I maintained a balance between driving at an appropriate speed and ensuring a smooth journey. The mum kept on asking me if her baby would be OK, and I was confident I knew the answer, but couldn't bring myself to say it. "They are doing everything they can for her, we will be at the hospital soon," was all I could muster, without giving any false hope or delivering the fatal news to her.

The resuscitation team at the hospital made a valiant effort to do everything they could. I stayed until a decision was made, feeling invested in the patient given my connection to their family. The resuscitation team carried on for 45 minutes then made the final call. I will never, ever forget the scream the mum let out. It still haunts me to this day, four years on, and I have never heard anything like it since. As I stood there, transfixed, a nurse gently guided me away from the scene. It dawned on me that I had lingered, watching the family – cradling their baby swathed in a shawl – long after the nurses and doctors had provided them with some space. It was as if I had been in a trance, and only when alerted to it did I notice tears streaming down the faces of the nurses, hidden from the family's view.

I drove back to the ambulance station in silence.

Andy McKinlay
Paramedic
Ambulance Services

Echoes of loss

The piercing shriek of grief,
Echoes still in the mind,
After years, it can be heard as clear as day,
The memory is not confined.

Now as old as they will ever be,
A husk of a person on the ground,
Still like a statue, one can't help but see,
The noise erupts, as if all around.

The sound of a broken heart,
As they watched a loved one depart,
A parent or child's mournful cry,
A bid of a final goodbye,

It rends through halls and gardens,
Rumbles 'cross roads and fields,
It grips your core, its power unhardened,
A haunting sound that never yields.

An unexpected moment,
The pain of loss and strife,
It comes suddenly and without intent,
A reminder of the fragility of life.

The shriek of grief, a sound so unique,
Each one a little different, yet all feel the same,
A memory that makes a soul feel weak.
Even after all these years, its impact will never fade away.

Matthew Herbert
Senior Clinical Advisor (Paramedic)
Emergency Care

Perfectly formed yet incredibly tiny

I remember this like it was yesterday.

It was a November night shift; I was crewing an ambulance with another (very new) paramedic. In the early hours of the morning, we were dispatched to an emergency call – category 1[5]: cardiac arrest. On the way, it was updated to, simply, "maternity". Our dispatcher radioed us, informing us the caller was ten years old, and they had called as their mum was in active labour. However, they couldn't ascertain whether or not the baby had been born yet.

We pulled up at the address at the same time as a team leader. Unsure what we would actually find, between the three of us we took all the equipment to prepare for any eventuality. The flat was several flights up, without a lift. Easier to take it now, than regret not having it once we were there. No sooner had we walked into the flat than we heard the cry of a newborn. Finding the mother, panicked, she told us she was 25 weeks pregnant, expecting twins. Our team leader requested another ambulance from control, and I watched as mum scooped her new baby into her arms. I couldn't get over just how tiny he was. When the next contraction came, she passed him to me – he fitted perfectly into the palm of my hand. She told us his name. We knew we needed to keep him as warm as possible, and thankfully our maternity pack is kitted for this – though the little hat and blanket made him look smaller still.

The sound of sirens from the second crew arriving echoed below us. The second twin was showing no sign of arrival just yet. Practically, we wouldn't be able to travel with both twins, her older child and the mother – there was just not enough room in the ambulance to safely transfer three patients, plus enough paramedics to see to each of them. We also knew we wouldn't be able to keep a small baby warm enough, for long enough, and there was no telling what condition the second twin would be in. We agreed with the mother, whose labour was progressing again, that we would take the first twin to the hospital, leaving our team leader on scene with the second ambulance waiting for baby number two. They'd all meet us there.

Alone in the back of the ambulance with this fragile new life, fear gripped me. Would he suddenly stop breathing? Born prematurely, he was perfectly formed yet incredibly tiny. I couldn't allow my inner turmoil to show. With limited equipment to keep him warm – just a blanket and a hat – I did the only thing I could: I talked to the baby throughout the journey to the hospital. I chatted about football, the passing scenery outside as the ambulance raced along, anything and everything to keep myself composed and reassure him that he wasn't alone. I prayed he'd be with his mum soon.

James Grant
Paramedic
Ambulance Services

Stress

I'm often asked about how stressful it is to be a paramedic.

It is, but not for the reasons you may think. Attending to patients in critical condition, where every moment counts, isn't what causes the stress. That's inherent in our job.

What truly adds to the stress is a system that inadvertently hinders our ability to provide care for patients. A system that leaves us waiting outside the hospital, unable to transfer our patients into hospital care due to a shortage of available beds. A system that sends us under emergency conditions to patients who don't actually need us... and so prevents us from attending the patients who do.

That's what makes it stressful.

Anonymous

Waiting

Tonight, the corridors bleed with people,
the radiators and lack of windows create a furnace,
fuelled by 20-degree heat.
The queue looks longer because social distance spreads out
   the seats,
the waiting is aggravating the impatient and irritated,
and the noise is stressing the hurting,
and our patients ask the same questions hour after hour,
"Do you really have to wait with us forever?"
Yes, we tell them, until you're handed over.

"But you must be missing so many emergencies –"
I've heard the same surprise in many voices,
It's a quote from a chorus of crowds and mixed ages.
But the break that's delayed due to high pressures,
and the desperate "is anyone available?" general broadcasts,[56]
and the late finishes.
Sometimes they're for someone who has drunk too much,
sometimes they're for a tiny cut,
or for the patient who wanted a non-existent wheelchair taxi
at four in the morning,
and the one whose family just needed help getting them
   out of the house.

Sometimes they're for the doctor whose patients need
   blue-light transport,
or for the patient who can't figure out the "total triage" system,
can't get past reception and the "you're number eleven",
Only to speak in that same voice when we call up, number
   twelve,
"You have to wait, too?"
We do.

Louise Sopher
Senior Paramedic and Resuscitation Practitioner
Ambulance Services

Christmas gifts

Christmas time is here
Torch and forceps on standby
Jimmy's got Lego

Christmas in the ambulance service

Black ribbons on white
Skodas skating through sleet – A
yellow Santa sleigh

Critical care

Sirens wailing. Blue
lights flashing. I smile and wave
as crit care drive by

Monica Thompson
Advanced Paramedic Practitioner (Urgent Care)
Ambulance Services

My first year

Paramedicine is a three-year degree. As part of the degree, we undertake practice placements in the ambulance service, as well as other clinical settings. In that time, I dealt with some truly horrific things. The one that stuck with me the most was the three-year-old boy feeding ducks. His grandmother had turned away for a few seconds and he was taken by the freezing river. We spent half an hour searching the banks until a police officer found him face down, over a kilometre downriver. He died later in hospital. I still struggle with that little boy's face today, seared into my mind. Thankfully, mercifully, things like this are rare and I went to nothing so terrifying as this in the rest of my degree.

So when I qualified as a paramedic, I was in for a hell of a surprise. Twenty-four weeks of a year working supernumerary on an ambulance crew was a distant dream when given the cold shock of full clinical responsibility. But hey, I'd had the necessary experience, I'd passed the exams, I knew the skills. I could do this. The thing is, in the NHS, there are few roles so isolating as paramedic practice in the ambulance service. In various regions, there are typically knowledgeable and resourceful individuals just a phone call away: a supportive team leader, a hospital unit, GPs, and believe me, a skilled dispatcher can often offer solutions to more challenges than you might imagine. But in the end, it's just you. In my NHS ambulance trust, most of my crewmates aren't paramedics or ambulance nurses and so the clinical responsibility is mine and mine alone.

Just several weeks out on my own after qualifying, I attended an asthmatic cancer patient who couldn't breathe. He was just skin and bones, 5-foot-nothing and the panic and pain he was in were carved on his face like a sculpture. It wasn't asthma – he was suffering from a spontaneous tension pneumothorax:[51] a medical presentation that is so inexplicably rare (around 7 in 100,000, I later learned), we expect only to see pneumothoraces caused by trauma. Still grappling with the disbelief that I was facing this situation, I found myself hastily performing a thoracocentesis –

stabbing his chest with a needle – while urging my crewmate to race to the hospital as quickly as possible. I was gripped with terror at the thought of him dying on me. He lived – though given his terminal cancer, I don't know how long for. Paramedics get very little, if any, feedback about the outcomes of patients we've attended. There is often no way to tell if you did well or badly, if they recovered or worsened, lived or died. So, I decided that he recovered and went home, and enjoyed his remaining time with his family.

A few months later, we're driving back to base for our half-hour meal break when an unmarked police car screams past on sirens. I didn't think much of it until less than a minute later we're dispatched to a category 1[5] call for a cardiac arrest, with the note underneath it: "hanging". We see the unmarked car again outside a well-manicured house in an affluent area of the town. We find the patient had clearly been dead for a little while, his feet turned purple from the gravity pull of blood. I fumbled and mumbled through my first suicide, filling out the recognition of life extinct[2] form as I went. One of those times I was so glad to have a team leader over the phone, guiding me through the process. We paid our respects, passed on his details to his GP and signed it all off and returned to base for a cup of tea and food. Welfare break.

At three o'clock in the morning, faced with a critical post-partum haemorrhage, a severely ill child, or a major trauma – when it's just me, my ambulance, and the urgent need for an immediate decision – I am starkly reminded of how isolated I am from immediate assistance. While I've been told that it gets easier with time and experience, I find that's not the case, especially during the first year.

Henry Thomas-Foy
Paramedic
Ambulance Services

Not just a driver

This is a brief poem I composed to shed light on some of the challenging scenarios that paramedics encounter, as well as the trauma we must navigate. We are more than mere drivers, a label all too often ascribed to us.

> My eyes are tired, my body aches, over 8 hours in and still no break.
>
> The call comes in, I drive to the scene,
> Weaving through traffic, blue light flashing, another victim has taken a bashing.
>
> He's hit her again, this time to a pulp,
> I see her face, I gasp, I gulp.
> No time to fear – she is in a bad way; she may not last another day.
>
> We do our best to keep her alive, despite our efforts she won't survive.
>
> Just another trauma to file away,
> Shake it off for another day.
>
> Another victim that wasn't a survivor, but I carry on as just an "ambulance driver".

Nicola Bromell-Pitter
Paramedic
Ambulance Services

A bit of a high...

I was working a nightshift as a paramedic as part of the Red Arrest Team[52] – or RAT – responding to cardiac arrests and serious trauma in the Hull and East Yorkshire region. After checking my vehicle and booking out drugs, I was alerted to my first job... backing up a crew at a cardiac arrest. Unphased, I made my way to the location. This was the bread and butter of my role.

As I arrived on scene, I could see the ambulance crew through the open front door of the bungalow performing chest compressions in the hallway. I integrated myself into the team to secure the patient's airway to enable successful ventilation, whilst the crew maintained effective chest compressions. The patient was in a VF.[6] He'd already had one shock from the defibrillator prior to my arrival, and at the next check he was still in VF. Shocked again, intravenous access[26] gained. Continued CPR. Expecting to shock again at the next two-minute check, we found his heart was now beating in an organised rhythm. We checked his breathing. He was making attempts to breathe by himself. Not resting on our laurels, we moved onto the post-ROSC[3] protocol to quickly assess and stabilise the patient in readiness for transfer to hospital. He continued to improve, and we moved him to the ambulance and put in a pre-alert to the hospital to have the resuscitation team meet us. Travelling in with the crew, he was starting to show an increasing level of consciousness by the time we handed him over to the hospital team. The prognosis for a good recovery was high, and we all felt satisfaction at a job well done. I led a quick hot debrief with the crew to ensure all were OK, and give congratulations all round, before radioing control to advise I was clear and available for any other 999 calls.

I didn't have to wait long before I was sent to a report of an unconscious female in her eighties at a care home. I was first on scene and, loaded with my response bags and defibrillator, I followed the carer to the patient's bedroom. She lay on the bed, emaciated and still. The carer passed me a lilac form with Do Not Attempt Resuscitation written in bold at the top. Checking that the form was valid (signed by a medical doctor), I radioed control to advise that no further resources would be required and began completing the necessary paperwork for the police and coroner.

After a quick cuppa back at the station, control alerted me to another job – a witnessed cardiac arrest in a pub. I arrived shortly after the crew and after battling through a scene of chaos with drinkers impeding my way, I found our patient and the crew in the corner of the pub. A member of the public had recognised that the collapsed male was in cardiac arrest and had started CPR while instructing someone else to call 999. Once again, this patient was in VF and after five shocks[53] we got a ROSC.[3] Whilst we'd been treating the patient, the pub had been cleared of drinkers by the police and we had a straight line outside to the ambulance, and on to the hospital for continuing care.

After two successful resuscitations I was on a bit of a high. It's good to know that sometimes we have a good outcome.

With an hour left of my shift I was starting to think I might just get off on time... nope, it wasn't to be, as my radio alerted me to another job. A six-week-old baby not breathing. The adrenaline kicked in and any thought of tiredness evaporated. As I pulled up outside the address, I saw the mother holding her baby tightly to her chest through the front window of the living room. I was aware of an ambulance crew parking on the road behind me as I walked through the front door and into the living room. I could see straight away that the baby was floppy in mum's arms. She didn't want to let go of her baby, sobbing with such deep emotion, I felt my stomach drop. I could see the baby had blue lips; they weren't breathing. I recall having to prise the baby from the mum's arms at the same time as telling her we were there to help the baby. Confirming cardiac arrest, as a team the crew and myself ventilated the baby with a paediatric bag-valve-mask[54] and started chest compressions. We placed paediatric defibrillator pads onto the baby's chest and back, our monitor showing us a thin green line. Asystole.[55] No electrical activity, no heartbeat. We did everything we could as we carried on CPR in the ambulance, the mum's sobs never abating, her eyes never leaving her baby's face.

I was finishing my paperwork in the reception of the emergency department when I heard the moment the consultant paediatrician told the mother her baby had died. A deep, guttural wail of hopelessness and misery reverberated down the cold, clinical corridors. I knew the prognosis had been poor for the baby, but I always have hope. *I don't want to do this job any more*, I thought. The high that I'd had from the previous successes of the night had gone, and a wave of despair swept over me.

I don't remember finishing my shift after that, but I do remember walking straight into my children's bedrooms when I got home, to check that they were OK.

Being a paramedic is the best job in the world... and sometimes the absolute worst.

Steve Johnson
Paramedic
Ambulance Services

Iron in the air

I wasn't long in the service and roughly a month off the training truck. I was working at one of the stations in the suburbs of the city with another Australian paramedic who had been in the service a few years. It was a Sunday night going into a Monday morning, and we had stopped at one of the smaller stations for a bathroom break. Over the radio, I heard control issue a general broadcast[56] for a road traffic collision[39] nearby. Since moving to the city, I'd been a bit of a "white cloud",[57] so I agreed we should report our availability, expecting a small fender bender with minimal to no injuries. It turns out we weren't far away and got to the scene within a few minutes.

Blue lights merged with the orange of the streetlights to illuminate a small crowd of people and a car on one side of the road. The police had already arrived and were walking towards the crowd as our ambulance pulled up. Through the knot of people in front of us, I could make out a figure prone on the ground. I took in the angle of his arms and legs, a pool of darkness that I knew would be blood gathering at his head. Nothing will ever prepare you for seeing a body, a person, like that. *He's fucked*. I made eye contact with my crewmate as they radioed control for assistance and I upgraded my facemask and grabbed an apron and gloves, both of which I hastily pulled on as I walked over to the patient. We were in the fourth wave of the COVID-19 pandemic, and I was well used to donning PPE on the move by now.

He was face-down with his head to one side, his breathing was slow, about four breaths a minute. His right arm was bent in a manner it should not have been, both legs angled unnaturally away from each other. I took his head in my hands, applying a manual manoeuvre to open his airway, and waited for my crewmate to join me. With the help of the police, we rolled the patient over – making an effort to preserve his airway and avoid further injury to his spine. One of the police supported me to manage the patient's airway, passing me equipment as my crewmate assessed the extent of his bleeding. I later found out it was that police officer's first day, one to remember, maybe not one he would want to. My apron didn't last long, having ripped on the rough surface of the road as we turned the patient over. I generally found them more of a hindrance than a help, so this was no great loss to me. We did what we are trained to do, muscle memory from the hours of simulation at university set in; we secured his airway, we breathed for him while he couldn't, we ascertained the extent of the damage, we obtained his observations (they didn't look good), we gave instructions to the police for more equipment from the truck: splints for his pelvis and limbs, the bag which held equipment to gain intravenous access[26] and administer the life-saving medicines that can help stop his bleeding.

For a long time, it was just me and my crewmate, observed by a self-declared close friend who held vigil by his side, the silence broken by the air being pushed into the patient's lungs by the bag-valve-mask.[54] The sirens were quiet at first, getting louder as they got closer, their lights mixing with the blue haze that already surrounded us.

The angels in orange, HEMS,[41] had finally arrived on scene. They quickly took over control of the patient's care and had me continue to give ventilation. Counting in my head, 1, 2, 3, 4, 5, 6 squeeze, 1, 2, 3, 4, 5, 6, squeeze. It was all I could do. We had done all we could, all I could do now was keep breathing for him. I watched as the HEMS doctor made incisions either side of the patient's chest, trying to release any air trapped inside. Another put a central line[31] in his femoral artery to get a better reading of his pulse. After this was completed, they gently moved me over to place an advanced airway, which would breathe for him and free me from ventilating him. I watched as they checked blood products between each other, ready to administer. Once set up, we reviewed the patient as a team. His observations weren't good – he'd lost a lot of blood – but was he past the point of no return? It was enough to transport him to the nearest major trauma centre. The HEMs doctor and paramedic jumped into the back of the ambulance with me. I could feel my heart beating fast as I heard the sirens ringing in the air, the lights bouncing along the streets in the dark. We all watched the machine breathe for the patient as we travelled, willing there to be a small improvement in his observations. A crowd of doctors and nurses were awaiting our arrival at the hospital, and assisted us to transfer the patient to a bed in the resuscitation bay. Then everyone was still and silent as the HEMS doctor gave the handover: clear, short and concise. Then, a hive of activity as the emergency department doctor issued instructions for her team to reassess and continue to treat the patient.

Retrieving our trolley bed, we started the clean-down process. The truck was a mess, equipment and plastic wrapping all over the place, blood pooling on the floor, the smell of iron in the air. My trousers had red stains at the knees, where I had been kneeling next to the patient's head as it oozed blood. We'd need to return to our station to restock, and to change uniform. I started the paperwork and began to go over everything we had done, reliving the job second by second to document it.

As I was leaving, I saw the friend outside the hospital doors, his forehead creased in worry. He asked where he could wait, and I took him to the relatives' room. As we walked down the hall, he turned to me and asked what he should tell the patient's girlfriend; was there any hope? I inhaled deeply, considering what to say to someone who, less than two hours earlier, had been casually walking to a party with their friend, only for a speeding car to veer off the road, striking their friend and propelling them over 10 metres. What do you say to a person who is put in an unenviable position of having to send a message none of us want to receive about a loved one? I felt hopeless in that moment. What could I say to him to offer comfort without offering false reassurance?

"Tell them to get here when they can but not to put themselves in danger doing so. I can't say what will happen, but someone will be out as soon as possible to give you an update." Those words sound so hollow.

This job is like riding a rollercoaster with a blindfold; you never know where the next turn is, you never know when you are going to feel your stomach drop. But that's the thrill of the job, never knowing what's going to happen next and having to react to the situations quickly. Not all jobs end the way we want, and often we don't even know the outcome of the patient. Is it better to know or not? Whatever the outcome, I take pride in my work and comfort in knowing I do all I can to help. I wouldn't change my job for anything in the world.

Emma Jane Briggs
Paramedic
Ambulance Services

Camaraderie

In the land where sirens wail,
and lights flash through the night's dark veil,
we share a jest, a knowing grin,
as fellow travellers in the din.

Through city streets and country lanes,
we ply our trades through sun and rain,
and as our paths will often cross,
we greet each other with a toss –

A friendly wave after a fleeting glance.
In passing, we share a dance,
but oftentimes, to our chagrin,
we find that it is not our kin.

For in the blur of lights and sound,
a Morrisons' van may be found.

And I wonder if there's Morrisons' drivers who
accidentally wave at ambulances too.[58]

Georgette Eaton
Consultant Paramedic
Ambulance Services

The shifts roll together

Three a.m. The radio alarms. There is a two-hour blue-light transfer – a four-hour return trip. It is too early in the shift to argue, but too late to feel safe. The patient needs a lung transplant and a space has become available at a specialist centre – how can I argue with that?

The road is dull, dark, and persistent. I roll down the window. I turn up the FM radio. I think my time-tested methods of remaining alert are working, yet every time my own radio makes a sound or there is a general broadcast,[56] my heart skips a beat. I can't work out if I am tired or just afraid of becoming sleepy. Stay awake.

There is a certain understanding among night-shift workers – we see a world hidden from those asleep: your empty bins, flung into the road by the wind, now upright and returned to the pavement so we can roll past. Your driveways which sparkle with ice – trust me, it was worse overnight – as we try to wheel your poorly relative into the ambulance. Finally, the full moon, and the pursuant evening dread.

A flurry of snow lands on the windscreen. The whiteout is now an eerie blue from our lights. Speed is pointless – I can't reach it and still see. I switch off the emergency lights and revert to normal road conditions. Danger versus safe progress. Sometimes the training is so clearly recalled.

My family ask what the worst thing is that I have seen. They, like friends and strangers, expect my reply to focus around blood and gore. But it isn't. It's death. Dead people, in states that we shouldn't expect to see them, when they should be buried or cremated. It is the utter dismay of the human condition – it's loneliness in those who dread Christmas, the capacity we have as humans to self-neglect or neglect others, to assume our neighbours are fine (because we cannot live forever worrying), or to turn a blind eye altogether. It's the truth, even on my days off, I see first-hand that the tale of the good Samaritan is more than just a story – it's reality. But it's also the 'granny dumping' season, when relatives reach the limits of their empathy. It's the lack of imagination for what is happening behind closed doors when all people see is an ambulance blocking their exit, and all they feel is their own anger. It's the way ambulances are now so commonplace that we are no longer a surprise on the road on blues, yet a fire engine pulling out of the same station seems to be capable of stopping time. It's the sad hilarity of the human condition that means that the call volume drops during a World Cup final, only to return to high pressures immediately after.

My crewmate can recognise the hospital from the intensity of the potholes as we enter. I hear him tell the patient that these are the last few bumps. The patient, meanwhile, groans about how uncomfortable the ambulances are. I allow them to joke that it is my driving. Maybe it really is.

Our next patient is unhappy about the wait, and states he pays his taxes. I used to respond: "Me too". Now I say, "Well good, otherwise we would have to let the police know". At least the wait for ambulances is more publicised now, its causes more accurately perceived – not a single factor can explain everything.

No one asks about the best moments in this work, only the gore or whether the media are right that we go to people who have an object stuck in various human orifices (we do). There are nice things, too: the dog who lures unsuspecting ambulance crews to his address by pressing his owner's pendant alarm when they are out because doing so means cuddles on emergency response and the slightly earlier return of the owner. Or the way we are all so invested in our uniqueness that we each hear the same conspiracy theory from patient after patient about the spread of COVID. Annoying, perhaps, but each theory is told with the same passion and enthusiasm that it is as if each person believes they are the only storyteller in the world, the first to discover this, therefore we must not have heard it before. This story has a lesson: people are more alike than they realise.

"How much further?" the tax-paying patient asks.

From the back of the ambulance, I look out the windows. I try to peer through the front, but it is so hard to see anything that meaningfully gives our location through the tiny bulkhead window. On station later, my crewmate thinks I can fit through that narrow gap that leads to the front in the old ambulances. They discuss this idea loudly from the room next door – I don't think they know I'm listening.

We arrive at hospital in the daytime, and the infection control nurse tells us they are unhappy with the fact we are wearing our jackets as we walk through the hospital corridor. But outside it is freezing, and I need a few minutes to adjust to the warmth of the emergency department.

In COVID's winters it was, of course, different. Then, it became acceptable to wear layers of plastic and zip a white suit over our uniforms. COVID was a beast that created its own etiquette. Daily, the rules changed, and with such vigour that it was as if we couldn't get anything right. Daily, it felt, we were told we had the wrong PPE: upgrade, downgrade – why are you wasting kit? We over-used our PPE on suspected COVID patients who were not overly symptomatic, finding ourselves raising our shoulders in discomfort beneath the plastic aprons when we stood in flats with multiple family members who were all unwell.

There. The silence. The knowledge we shared when we watched the young, the staff, or anyone not expected to be so unwell with a virus, who we were about to blue-light to hospital. There – the raised eyebrows and widened eyes as we looked at each other, a silent phrase shared: are you OK? The same knowledge shared when attending to elderly fallers who, at five in the morning, needed lifting from the floor with the same arms that (though cleaned) had guided the COVID patient out of their house and the same uniform exposed around the gaps in the apron when that patient coughed. Yet somehow, we were, in your perception, safer than walking into hospital.

My crewmate has parked the old Mercedes on a steep driveway. The steps have become a ship's ladder (for those of us who are short, anyway), only my feet land on concrete rather than the sea to explore. There is another home to enter, another patient to see. This time it's muscular back pain. Next time it's a chronic cough. After that, it's tooth pain (how did that get through to us?); then finger pain; cellulitis; blood in a catheter. Nosebleeds – small and large. Vagueness – really, that should be a diagnosis. Panic attacks; hallucinations; discharged home but can't mobilise; discharged home but can't eat; discharged home but can't take medications. "Unconscious" – asleep. Patient with a lump that has already been diagnosed; throat pain; the world's smallest cut on a finger; shoulder dislocations.

Cardiac arrest.

Life's key moments are juxtaposed in one shift. We are no longer just an emergency service.

I have quit full-time work, partly because nights are approached senselessly. We're poached by every uncertainty. The uncertainties of the public, who seek reassurance. The uncertainties of the system, which cannot confidently make callers wait until social hours for problems that do not sound like emergencies (but could be). The uncertainties of our government, which has not funded an alternative for so many circumstances. The uncertainties of other systems, which cannot help a person up off the floor. The uncertainties of us all for the patients who don't know to tell us we are no longer needed after many hours, so we drive dozens of miles in the middle of the night, just in case, but find them well, asleep, and favouring a strong preference for dreamland over us.

The challenge lies in determining what constitutes a life-threatening situation when there isn't someone present to assess your condition or provide feedback on your appearance. Without access to objective observations or the ability to interpret medical history, it becomes even more difficult to gauge the severity of an injury, especially if it's your first experience with such an incident. Are our frustrations directed towards patients, or towards the shortcomings of our healthcare system? And how can we reform a system that inadvertently fosters this innate human desire for reassurance?

Click. The ambulance handbrake is finally raised. A high-pitched sound comes through the screen in the vehicle, accompanied by a red flashing message: end of shift. A half-smiling crew are approaching, their kit bags strung over their shoulders, ready to take over our ambulance for the day.

Time merges, the days blending into one another. Some jobs, whether "big" or not, are clear, and others long forgotten. Many of us leave but return to do some shifts, enough to feel we haven't entirely disconnected. Year after year, this is the job that persists, the foundation of a career and the part of the core that sometimes needs resolidifying. Is that what makes frontline work so enticing? If not just that, is it the colleagues, the social element, the patients, or the ability to see an area instead of just an office and its nearby streets? Or, perhaps, I wonder, is it the fact that its purpose is literally sewn into the logo and printed on our backs?

Louise Sopher
Senior Paramedic and Resuscitation Practitioner
Ambulance Services

That time we stumbled upon a stabbing

It was the cold pre-dawn in one of the more deprived areas of Birmingham, and my crewmate and I were preparing to convey a three-year-old child to hospital. She'd had a febrile convulsion[59] and had recovered well, but her temperature was still very high despite having both paracetamol and ibuprofen. We were concerned she may have an underlying infection, and would perhaps have another convulsion.

We made our way down the many flights of stairs of the tower block to the ambulance, buckling in the parents and seeing our patient was comfortable in readiness to navigate the quiet city roads. Jumping into the driver's seat and turning on the engine, my headlights illuminated the backs of other family members who had been supporting the parents of the patient in the flat, who were making their own way home. I was just about to release the handbrake, looking ahead as I gently applied the accelerator to pull away, when I noticed two of the relatives had stopped on the pavement, waving their arms frantically in the air towards me and pointing up ahead. I'd be driving past them to get to the main road anyway, so I rolled the ambulance to a stop as I approached them. As I got closer, my headlights illuminated some commotion just up ahead: a small group of young people wearing hoodies were bundled around a single person lying on the floor. It took a moment for me to register that they were hitting the prone individual with what looked like bats. The group momentarily froze in my headlights, then fled in different directions into the estate. I told the relatives to get into their cars or homes, quickly, and lock their doors.

I called through to my colleague in the back of the ambulance, "There's something going on out here, I'm just going to go and take a look". I pulled up on the side of the road, hand poised on the radio on my belt as I walked over, alert for any movement in my peripheral vision as I approached the single person writhing in the road. No older than a teenager, the headlights of the ambulance were reflected in the whites of his eyes as he gasped

"I'VE BEEN STABBED! I'VE BEEN STABBED!"

I kneeled beside him and saw slashes in his clothes and a gaping wound to his thigh. What I thought were bats had in fact been machetes.

"I'm going to grab some equipment; I'll be right back."

I got on the radio as I ran to the back of the ambulance. We already had a patient on board who needed to attend hospital. Whilst they wouldn't need the same equipment my new patient would need, I would need help: "I need red backup and police," I panted into my handheld radio. "We've got a running call for a patient at our current location who has been stabbed. Is the critical care team available?"

I opened the ambulance door and jumped into the back, telling my crewmate the situation as I started to pull some kit together to take back outside. I clocked the little girl was blissfully asleep, her parents looking up at me quizzically. I'd need to leave it to my crewmate to explain the situation to them. My plan was to render first aid while we waited for back-up. Loaded with the equipment I thought I would need, I hesitated at the open door at the back of the ambulance before jumping down, wondering whether it was a stupid idea for me to go back out to the patient alone, given he'd just been stabbed. I often find myself returning to this moment of uncertainty whenever I reflect on this job, pondering whether I would have made the same decision had the subsequent moment not occurred.

I heard a scream: "HE'S GOT A MACHETE!"

Automatically, I dropped the kit where I was standing in the back of the ambulance, pulled the door shut and locked us in. The first rule of first aid: danger, protect yourself. I can't help anyone if I'm injured.

I peered out of the small window on the side of the ambulance. I could see the patient lying on the floor, still writhing, no large pool of blood had formed around him. Where my headlights had emptied the road initially, a crowd was gathering around the figure on the floor, standing around. I strained to see any weapons in their hands, aware of my heart beating rapidly against my ribs – I was no longer willing to approach alone. My crewmate and I talked about what to do. We decided we couldn't go over until the police arrived and continued to watch through the small opening of the window. I updated our control whilst my crewmate talked to the parents of the child, reassuring them that we were safe with the doors locked. Now locked in the back of the ambulance, I couldn't drive us away. We were stuck there until more help arrived.

We were all jolted by a bang on the side of the ambulance, followed by a shout: "YOU NEED TO DO SOMETHING, HE'S BEEN STABBED, HE COULD DIE."

I replied through the small opening on the window, my voice sounding much calmer than I felt; "We have a child in the ambulance, we have called for another ambulance, it won't be long."

It didn't appease him. I feel an enormous pang of guilt. Watching through the window, I could see the patient becoming increasingly still. Emotion was mounting up inside me, mentally begging "Police please, please, come soon please I need to get over there". Each second that ticked by was agonisingly slow.

A new noise, a woman's wail, came from the front of the vehicle. I looked out, seeing an older woman with another youth, the gang of youths surrounding the patient on the floor thinning out. "Please. My son has been stabbed. Please, you need to do something," my heart tugged as she begged. Control updated us that a second ambulance crew was nearby, and the police had been requested.

With our first patient sleeping soundly, her observations remaining stable since our initial attendance, my crewmate and I agreed with the parents that we would like to help the person outside. They understood the gravity of the situation, the empathy of the mother palpable as she told us to help someone else's child.

Splitting the equipment between us, my crewmate and I updated control that we were going to make contact with the patient now, believing his condition to have deteriorated. "We're coming now," I told the mother as we walked briskly to her son in the road. I explained to her that we already had a small child on board who we were taking to hospital when we came across her son. It did not appease her, telling me in reply simply that her son is 16. Approaching the patient, we found the atmosphere had changed to one of respect and concern; the youths standing around as if in a vigil, two kneeling beside our patient.

I had an inward sigh of relief finding him still conscious. With the bystanders forming a ring, the mother, my crewmate and I with the patient in the inner circle, we cut off his clothes – talking to him as we assessed the damage. He had multiple large gaping wounds across the entire length of his torso, and a particularly deep wound to his thigh which I'd spotted initially. There must have been more than ten wounds, all bleeding, but thankfully none significantly. However, with a stab wound, there is no telling what the underlying damage could be – he was still very much a critical patient. We started applying pressure to the wounds, starting with the gaping wound on the thigh – which was bleeding more than the others, and I was aware of its proximity to the femoral artery – before moving back to those on the torso, double checking that these had not caused further damage to his lungs. My crewmate worked systematically, applying oxygen and preparing to gain intravenous access.[26]

Blue lights illuminated the scene – the second ambulance and several police cars arrived in succession. I breathed a sigh of relief as a paramedic I knew well approached us, our ring of bystanders parting to let her through. She had the critical care team on the radio and handed it to me – they were 20 minutes away. I know my city, and I knew we were 10 minutes away from the trauma centre. I remember a conference talk I attended a few years ago, where a consultant in emergency medicine told us that patients who have been stabbed don't need to be in the back of an ambulance, they don't even need to be in the resuscitation area in the emergency department, they need to be in theatre. I told the team over the radio that we were not waiting, we would convey to the trauma centre immediately. The critical care paramedic on the radio agreed this sounded like the best option, and we prepared the patient to be transported to hospital. The other crew agreed to take our original patient to the children's hospital.

Blue lights illuminated the streets in the growing dawn as we drove on emergency conditions to the trauma centre, the patient remaining stable during the journey as we continued to treat his pain and administer medicines that pre-empt his blood loss. We made the hospital aware of our impending arrival, and a trauma team greeted us at the entrance. The handover was smooth, and we transferred the patient to their bed and their care – his mum never far away from him.

I sat writing my paperwork in reception, my heart still bounding ten to the dozen as the adrenaline wore off. My crewmate brought me a cup of tea, which I sipped gratefully between writing my notes. Our operational manager arrived, and we had a short debrief. I relayed the details, trying to make sense of everything that had just happened, wondering if I had done the right thing, whether I should have gone back over with the kit straight away like I said I would, remembering the pain and displeasure in his mother's eyes as she asked us for help.

I'll always be conflicted when I think back to this job. If someone hadn't shouted there was still a person with a machete nearby, I would have been with the patient alone. Should I have been? Could I have been injured? What would we have done if the little girl we had on board already was more unwell, and needed immediate treatment in hospital, or even resuscitation? In our case, the child was conveyed to the children's hospital and was well, and the teenager who had been stabbed survived. I have to remember that these real outcomes are what matter the most. But the question I ask myself remains, had the situation been any different, who would have mattered more?

Lucy McKenzie
Paramedic
Ambulance Services

itsokaynottobeokay

As I write this story, I look around. I am surrounded by colleagues who spend their working days trying to help others. These very same people are battling their own demons whilst delivering care and compassion in sometimes impossible circumstances. Endless jobs stack on the screens, which we have no hope of ever clearing. People are dying. Our patients are dying because there aren't enough of us, because our services are so stretched.

I open a letter addressed to me. It comes as no surprise. A paramedic with over 30 years' experience has written his resignation. This is the fifth resignation in as many months. That's over a hundred years of clinical experience gone...

poof

Just like that. It's irreplaceable.

As I navigate the empty city streets at 4 a.m., memories flow into and out of my mind. I choose not to fight them; I allow them to come and go like the tide being drawn by the brightest moon.

One memory leads to another and, although they are completely unrelated, they flow seamlessly together. The man hanging in the outbuilding; the bodies entwined in the twisted metal of the crashed car; the smell of burnt flesh in the house fire; the taste of a mother's milk on the lips of her tiny baby delivered early at home; and the feeling of a dying brain as my fingers feel the boggy mass of a crushed skull. A smell can take me back instantly to a situation that I would give almost anything to forget. All of my senses are overwhelmed in the flood of these memories, but I grip the steering wheel and I remember to breathe.

It must have been six or seven years ago now, when I walked into the bathroom and saw a woman hanging. I immediately thought my 999 career was over. I was not OK. Fast forward to now, it seems to be generally acceptable to admit that #itsokaynottobeokay. Despite that, it can still be such a taboo subject to discuss. Maybe it's time to accept that we really are all a little bit broken, but that's OK. We're broken together. I can't help but ponder whether any of my late colleagues, who succumbed to their inner demons, would have opted for a different path had they experienced the level of acceptance that exists today.

As I drive alone at night, I can see faces of patients in the bushes as I speed by, illuminated by my blue lights.

I see dead people.

Apparently, that's perfectly normal. It's a normal reaction to an abnormal situation. Your brain is trying to process the information it has been given. It replays in our waking hours in the form of flashbacks or intrusive memories and invades our sleep with nightmares and fear. It's perfectly normal.

I do wish it would fuck off though. I've got work to do.

Nic Haywood
Paramedic
Ambulance Services

Heather

Curled up on the bedroom floor
She waits, still as a rock
The stillness only broken
By the tick of the mantlepiece clock

Her fragile frame unable to rise
Empty rooms echo with the sound of her pleas
Lying alone in the darkness
She pulls her nightdress over her knees

Streaks of blue light slice through net curtains
And pour across the tired walls
The muffled sound of voices and boots
A gust of dawn air fills the hall

Kneeling down on threadbare carpet
Working through the whats and whys
I'm drawn to the evidence on the walls
Memories of the years gone by

I glance at photos of their halcyon days
Shoulder to shoulder in a smoky cloud
Barrel glasses on a varnished table
Faces turned pale from the camera flash in the crowd

Lounging in deck chairs on the beach
Their smiles warmed by the afternoon sun
Next to snapshots of polished moves in dance halls
Holding hands, waltzing and waiting to be spun

She searches the corners of her mind
To tell us of their love story
These thoughts bring life back to a face
That had long forgotten about glory

They met in a factory years ago
Making munitions and shells
A simple life together full of joy
Until he said his final farewell

She unfolds her legs and gets to her feet
Her night on the floor now over
Burgundy slippers shuffle side by side
As frail hands pull a cardigan round bony shoulders

Her silhouette fades behind frosted glass
To another day chalking off the hours
The house now silent and still
She gets on with her day, and we ours

Under scarlet skies I make my way home
To a house filled with memories of my own
"Good day?" she asks, as I pull off my boots
And suddenly I'm eclipsed,

By a momentary flash of cognisance
That our time is finite and flies
I need to stop and take notice
And look into her blue–green eyes

To remember every detail and line
Time will overtake us, no longer together
Stoically shuffling alone
like Heather.

Anonymous

The break of day

As a paramedic, I've been privileged to witness both the darkest and most inspiring aspects of human nature, creating countless memories, some of which I've kept to myself, unshared with family or friends. While there are numerous stories I could recount, I've chosen to focus on just one.

Working as a paramedic practitioner on a solo response car often meant I was sent to many patients who were receiving palliative care or were approaching the end of their life. One of my proudest moments was one of these calls.

It was a week before Christmas, and the night freezing. I was on my last of four consecutive night shifts, and it was hectic. It was 6:30 a.m., and my shift finished at seven. I had just sat down in the mess room with a hot cup of tea when my radio went off. I was being sent to a 45-year-old female with breathing difficulties. I'll always remember this job for so many reasons. She lived in a remote country cottage that was in the middle of nowhere. The drive to the job, up all these dark, narrow country roads in the cold with a dense and low fog, was really eerie. More Halloween vibes than Christmas cheer.

I was met at the door by the patient's family. The concern for her current condition was tangible, and I could see their eyes were red from crying. I knew from the get-go that this would be one of those jobs that would be significant in some way. We can all relate to that feeling – that feeling in your gut that you can never really explain to others who don't share in your experience in the emergency services. As I entered the front room, I could see a hospital bed and various other hospital paraphernalia: a syringe driver, a fluid stand, and a portable oxygen machine and a supply of oxygen cylinders. My patient was sitting up in bed, supported by at least four pillows. She was pale, sweaty, and working really hard to breathe. Despite the obvious effort to breathe, she greeted me with the warmest of smiles.

The house was roasting hot, so hot I thought I might faint. But she felt the cold. As I removed my coat and fleece, I listened to her story. She had stage three cancer and was for palliative care only. I recall feeling this overwhelming connection between us that I still can't really explain to this day. She showed me her advance care plan, clearly pointing out that she had a do-not-resuscitate order and she wanted to die at home. She then asked me to find a way to send her family out for a bit; she wanted to talk to me alone.

She was clearly exhausted. Whenever she was looking at me, I felt her eyes were boring me out and trying to send my soul a message. I had a keen sense I knew that she was trying to tell me something meaningful, without really saying it out loud. I could tell she had had enough of fighting and was giving up. I asked the family to give us a few minutes for me to get her a bit more settled, and when they left the room, she told me she was ready to die and that she thought it was happening now.

This is one of those situations where I always think that no university degree or training course can ever teach you what to do or how you will react in this moment. After all, no one ever becomes a paramedic not to help people, to make them better, with the hope you will save lives. From day one, we are drilled to react and treat our patients' medical issues. Yet, in end-of-life care, this takes on a different perspective and a deeper meaning. My traditional instincts told me to beg for an ambulance ASAP. But I had that feeling that even if they drove at the speed of light, they still couldn't get here in time.

My critical reasoning head kicked in, and I knew it was not what the patient wanted. Though I did offer it to her – even with an advance care plan in place, she had the right to change her mind. She didn't change her mind, and she didn't want me to call her palliative care team, as she didn't like the nurse who always came. I set to make her comfortable. I could see she was in pain, so I started working my way through administering her opiate pain relief, which was part of the anticipatory medicines pack prescribed by her hospice. This also eased the breathing but made it feeble and more laboured. I suggested it was time to bring her family back in, but she asked me not to. I recall this made me feel sad and a bit awkward. It must have shown on my face as she grabbed my hand and said she wanted to protect them. She didn't want the last memory of her being her choking for breath. She then said she trusted me and could tell I was a kind soul. I nodded in acknowledgement, trying not to choke on the lump I had in my own throat. I asked if there was anything else I could do for her. "Yes," she replied, and went on to explain that her daughter was getting married in a few months, and her son was expecting a baby in the next few weeks. She had planned to write them both letters, but she had not got the chance. She asked me if I could do it for her. I didn't hesitate to say yes; of course I would.

She directed me to where I could find all the paper and envelopes. I updated the control room: I was remaining on the scene as death was imminent. I then turned my radio down so it would not distract me at this moment, panicking that I would not be able to write quickly enough. I popped outside the door where the family was waiting and saw they had all fallen asleep on the sofa together. I was thankful for this, as I had no idea how I was going to explain that their mum and wife did not want them to be with her when she died. I returned, and she dictated a letter for her daughter to open on her wedding day, and then another to her son to open on the day his baby was born.

The time felt like it passed quickly, and when I looked up at the window, I could see the sun was coming up. My finish time had passed long ago. When I sealed the final envelope, I looked to see the dawn light catching her face. She just looked so peaceful. Her breathing was very shallow now, and her heart rate was slowing down. Almost sleepily, she smiled at me and thanked me for helping her. It had been my honour. I knew she was slipping away, and I asked if I could bring her family back in to be with her, explaining that I thought it was time. She nodded in agreement. I woke her family up, and we all returned to the room. Only this time, I kept my distance, giving her family the space to have those last few precious moments with her.

She passed away a few minutes later, just as day fully broke through, the sun now beaming down onto her in full. This was one of the most meaningful moments I have ever witnessed in my ambulance career. It brought so much comfort to her family; she had always loved the sun.

I thought about that job all the way home, and for many days after.

Several weeks later, during a day shift, I received a summons from my management team to return to the station, leaving me feeling anxious and uncertain about the reason behind the recall. As I made my way back to the station, my mind raced with apprehension. Upon entering the station, I was greeted by the sight of a family with a pram. It wasn't until I saw the father, beaming at me across the garage as I parked the car, that the pieces of the puzzle fell into place – this was the son of the woman for whom I had written a letter, dictated by her during her final moments the month before. He had come to express his gratitude personally for the support I had provided to his family and his mother during her final hours. Tears flowed freely as we embraced. Whilst I've saved many lives as a paramedic, supporting the death of this patient stands out as the proudest moment of my ambulance career.

Charley Beale
Advanced Care Practitioner (Paramedic)
Secondary Care

A guide for navigating the profession

Being a paramedic is a humbling experience, where the cycle of life unfolds before our eyes every shift, with moments of both new beginnings and farewells. I could share countless stories from my 25 years on the job, from the miraculous to the heart-breaking, but those tales are for another time. To those coming into this profession and reading this, you need a steady head, a warmth of spirit, and humility. But, whilst you'll bring your natural gifts and life experiences to these calls, don't be a hero: true strength and integrity stem from setting aside ego.

Finally, look after each other, talk and share your concerns, meet in the fresh air and enjoy the gift of laughter. Be active listeners, for together, we are a unique bunch of clinicians and in fostering camaraderie, we form a distinctive community working to provide care in the prehospital realm. Whether volunteers or professionals, take pride in your contributions.

Thank you for being the difference 24/7.

Adrian McGrath
Clinical Support Paramedic
Ambulance Services

ENDNOTES

1. *DATIX*: a risk management information system which gathers data on processes and errors. Responding appropriately when things go wrong is key to the NHS continuously improving the safety of patients.
2. *Recognition of life extinct (ROLE)*: confirmation that death has occurred. This is the first in a number of steps which need to be completed before the legal registration of death takes place. Paramedics can only verify the "Fact of Death". They cannot "Certify" the cause of death. Certification must be undertaken by a medical doctor.
3. *Return of spontaneous circulation (ROSC)*: the return of a sustained heart rhythm that perfuses the body after the heart has stopped. It is commonly associated with significant respiratory effort.
4. *Category 2*: classed as an emergency or a potentially serious condition that may require rapid assessment, urgent on-scene intervention and/or urgent transport.
5. *Category 1*: for people with life-threatening illnesses or injuries.
6. *Ventricular fibrillation (VF)*: a type of irregular heart rhythm (arrhythmia). During ventricular fibrillation, the lower heart chambers contract in a very rapid and uncoordinated manner. As a result, the heart does not pump blood to the rest of the body.
7. *Electrocardiogram (ECG)*: this is a reading of the electrical activity of the heart, measuring rate, rhythm and any irregularities. It can be used to diagnose heart attacks or conditions characterised by abnormal heart rhythm.
8. *Myocardial infarction (MI)*: the medical term for a heart attack.
9. *Percutaneous coronary intervention (PCI)*: this is a non-surgical procedure which treats blockages in a coronary artery. It opens up narrowed or blocked sections of the artery, restoring blood flow to the heart.
10. This poem originated from a light-hearted response to the common question, "Which one of you is the ambulance driver?" However, it evolved to capture the essence of our work as a crew on the road. It encapsulates the diverse range of incidents we respond to, the multitude of skills we acquire, and the support we offer to patients and their families. While witnessing the miracle of new life fills us with joy, it is equally heart-wrenching to witness life depart from this world.
11. *Cannulate*: the act of putting a thin tube into a part of the body. This term is often used synonymously with intravenous access (see note 25).
12. *Urinary tract infection (UTI)*: an infection of any part of the urinary system: kidneys, ureters, bladder and urethra.
13. *Auscultate*: to examine a patient by listening to sounds from the heart, lungs, or other organs, using a stethoscope.

14. *Category 3*: classified as urgent. These are problems (not immediately life-threatening) that need treatment to relieve suffering (e.g. pain control) and transport or clinical assessment and management at the scene.
15. *Tourniquet*: a device which applies pressure to a limb or extremity in order to stop the flow of blood.
16. *Varus*: a deformity in which an anatomical part is turned inward toward the midline of the body to an abnormal degree.
17. *Valgus*: a deformity in which an anatomical part is turned outward away from the midline of the body to an abnormal degree.
18. *Peripheral vertigo*: a symptom characterised by a false sensation of spinning or rotation of oneself or the surroundings. This occurs due to a problem in the part of the inner ear that controls balance.
19. *Category 4*: for incidents that are not urgent but need assessment (face-to-face or telephone), and possibly transport, within a clinically appropriate timeframe.
20. *BASICS doctor*: British Association for Immediate Care doctors are on call in their free time to provide direct clinical care and support to the most critically unwell patients.
21. *Hypovolaemia*: a condition that occurs when the body loses fluid, such as blood or water.
22. *Mobile data terminal (MDT)*: a computerised device used in the ambulance service to communicate with a central dispatcher in ambulance service control.
23. *Emergency care assistant (ECA)*: a type of emergency medical service worker who supports paramedics and drives ambulances under emergency conditions.
24. *Nebuliser*: a drug delivery device which administers medication in the form of a mist inhaled into the lungs. Nebulisers are commonly used in the treatment of respiratory disorders, such as asthma, where the drug can be absorbed directly by the lung tissue.
25. *Bronchodilator*: a type of medication which relaxes the muscles in the lungs and causes a widening of the passages which conduct air into the lungs.
26. *Intravenous access*: a technique in which a cannula is placed inside a vein to provide venous access to administer medicines or fluids.
27. Antihistamines are no longer part of the medication regime for acute anaphylaxis, but were in previous versions of UK ambulance services clinical practice guidelines.
28. *Unexploded ordnance (UXOs)*: bombs or explosive weapons which did not explode when they were employed and still pose a risk of detonation, sometimes many decades after they were used or discarded.
29. *Haemodynamics*: relating to the flow of blood within the organs and tissues of the body.
30. *Nasogastric tube*: a tube that is inserted through the nose, down the throat and oesophagus, and into the stomach.
31. *Central line*: a soft, flexible, hollow tube that is placed into a large vein, such as the superior vena cava.
32. *Analgesia*: medication that acts to relieve pain.

33. *ST elevation*: in electrocardiography, this represents the period when the cardiac ventricles are in a resting state between contracting and relaxing. ST elevation refers to a finding on an electrocardiogram where the trace in the ST segment is abnormally high above the baseline, indicating a lack of oxygen in the heart muscle, caused by a blockage in a blood vessel in the heart (a heart attack).
34. *HAZMAT suit*: an overall garment worn to protect people from hazardous materials or substances, including chemicals, biological agents or radioactive materials. These suits are commonly white in colour.
35. *N95 mask*: a respiratory protective mask designed to achieve a very close facial fit and to provide very efficient filtration of airborne particles. These were the standard masks issued to healthcare professionals during the COVID-19 pandemic.
36. *Health and Care Professions Council (HCPC) Guidelines*: the Health and Care Professions Council is an organisation which regulates health, psychological and care professionals in the United Kingdom. It sets standards, holds a register, quality assures education and investigates complaints. It also issues profession-specific guidelines that set out a professional standard of practice.
37. *Shit magnet*: a colloquial and superstitious expression referring to a person who, for some inexplicable reason, "attracts" bad jobs, such as patients with life-threatening conditions, trauma and death.
38. *Tonic-clonic seizure*: a loss of consciousness and violent muscle contractions. A type of seizure most people will recognise.
39. *Road traffic collision (RTC)*: otherwise known as a motor vehicle crash or a car crash.
40. *iGel*: a supraglottic airway device made by Intersurgical Ltd. Supraglottic airway devices facilitate ventilation and oxygenation without penetrating the vocal cords.
41. *Helicopter Emergency Medical Services (HEMS)*: a crew, typically made up of an emergency medicine doctor and a paramedic, who provide rapid response via helicopter.
42. *Critical care paramedics*: paramedics who are specialists in caring for patients with serious or major trauma, critical or complex acute illness and those requiring resuscitation.
43. *LifePak*: a brand of cardiac defibrillator produced by the medical technology company Physio-Control.
44. *EZ-IO*: a small device that functions like a traditional drill and drill bit, consisting of a reusable, battery-powered driver and disposable, hollow needle which enables the insertion of a needle into a bone for the delivery of medication in emergency situations. Used in particular when intravenous access cannot be obtained.
45. *Low-flow state*: where the heart is still beating, but is unable to produce a pulse due to insufficient blood volume.
46. *Intermittent positive pressure ventilation (IPPV)*: a respiratory therapy treatment for people who are breathing spontaneously, but slowly. The lungs are expanded by actively blowing air into them.

47. *Patency*: the state of being open, not blocked or obstructed.
48. *End-tidal CO$_2$*: the level of carbon dioxide released at the end of an exhaled breath, reflecting the patient's ventilatory status.
49. *Intravascular volume*: the volume of blood within a patient's circulatory system.
50. *Self-sustained perfusion*: the continuous flow of blood or fluid to tissues and organs.
51. *Spontaneous tension pneumothorax*: an abnormal condition of the lung characterised by the accumulation of gas in the space between the lungs and the chest wall. This condition occurs without an obvious cause.
52. *Red Arrest Team (RAT)*: a team composed of ambulance clinicians who have received training in leadership, advanced decision making and specific enhanced skills for managing patients in cardiac arrest.
53. *Shocks*: a colloquial term for the electrical pulses delivered by a defibrillator.
54. *Bag-valve-mask (BVM)*: a hand-held device commonly used to deliver breaths to patients who are not breathing or are not breathing adequately.
55. *Asystole*: the total cessation of electrical activity in the heart, resulting in no contraction of the heart muscle and no blood flow to the body.
56. *General broadcast*: an open-channel request made by ambulance control for ambulances to respond to unallocated 999 calls.
57. *White cloud*: a colloquial term that refers to someone who has had a streak of good luck, where patients aren't sick and where paramedic skills are often not needed.
58. We always wave to colleagues whenever we drive past each other at work. A longstanding joke among all UK ambulance services is the frequency with which we have waved at a Morrisons' van thinking it is another ambulance.
59. *Febrile convulsion*: a seizure that occurs in children aged between six months and six years when they have a high fever.